Diet for CROHN'S DISEASE, ULCERATIVE COLITIS, DIVERTICULITIS, CELIAC DISEASE, CYSTIC FIBROSIS and CHRONIC DIARRHEA

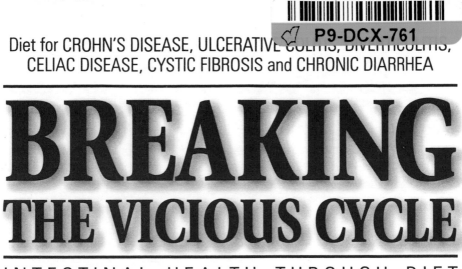

BREAKING
THE VICIOUS CYCLE

INTESTINAL HEALTH THROUGH DIET

Diet for CROHN'S DISEASE, ULCERATIVE COLITIS, DIVERTICULITIS, CELIAC DISEASE, CYSTIC FIBROSIS and CHRONIC DIARRHEA

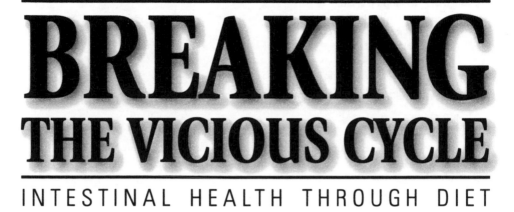

BREAKING
THE VICIOUS CYCLE

INTESTINAL HEALTH THROUGH DIET

Elaine Gottschall B.A.,M.Sc.

The Kirkton Press • Baltimore, Ontario, Canada

Copyright© 2010 Kirkton Press Limited

Published by: Kirkton Press Ltd.
                396 Grills Road
                RR #2
                Baltimore, Ontario
                Canada K0K 1C0
                www.breakingtheviciouscycle.info
                email: kirkton@eagle.ca

Printed and bound in Canada

Orders for additional copies of this book may be obtained through The Kirkton Press

Thirteenth Printing – May 2010

12 WC 07

Canadian Cataloguing in Publication Data
Gottschall, Elaine Gloria, 1921-2005
   Breaking the Vicious Cycle, Intestinal Health through Diet.

Rev. ed. of: Food and the Gut Reaction: Intestinal Health through Diet.
Includes bibliographical references and index.

ISNB 0-9692768-1-8

1. Intestines–Diseases–Diet Therapy
2. Inflammatory bowel diseases–Diet Therapy
I. Title. II. Title: Food and the Gut Reaction: Intestinal Health through Diet.

RC860.G67   1994   641.5'631   C94-931288-6

Cover Illustration – Marilyn Jones

ACKNOWLEDGEMENTS

In the research, writing, and publishing of this book I received moral, intellectual, and emotional support from many people. Among these, the following people stand out and to them goes my deepest appreciation:

Dr. Donald B. McMillan for his time, expertise, support, and friendship.

Catheryne Dahlke for her ability to establish order and coherence to the present reorganization of this book.

Patricia Wilson for her friendship and willingness to share her artistic talents by producing the illustrations.

Diane Jewkes for her patience and expertise in editing the manuscript.

Sue Brown, Callie Cesarini, Marge Moulton, Debbie Newsted, and Jane Sexsmith for their good humor and assistance in helping me execute the numerous revisions.

Valerie Tabone and Sandra Rule of the Department of Graphic Services (University of Western Ontario) for their cooperation and expertise in typesetting and artistic layout of the manuscript.

My husband, Herbert, for his unlimited patience, moral support, and continual prodding to "write the book." My daughter, Judith Lynn Herod, and her friend, Tad Crohn, for their superb job of initial editing.

My daughter, Joan Beth Gottschall, for her continual encouragement.

IMPORTANT NOTICE TO THE READER:

This book contains a diet and nutritional information that, in the author's experience, has helped those who have followed it.

The author recognizes that the treatment of illness and the enhancement of health through diet should be supervised by a duly qualified physician. Readers should not engage in self diagnosis and self treatment. Consult your doctor before starting the regimen proposed here. This book will be particularly complemented by discussions with a physician who has a particular interest or training in nutrition.

The author and publisher do not assume medical or legal liability for the use or misuse of the information and regimen contained in this book.

Publisher's Note:

The Internet is both friend and foe to those on the Specific Carbohydrate Diet™ (SCD). Friend, thanks to the support and information it offers; foe because it is so important to exercise care and, even, skepticism when researching the SCD on line.

The Internet abounds with food products and even versions of the diet claiming to be SCD legal, compliant or improved. Be very, very critical about what you read. Without talking directly to the manufacturer, it is impossible to know if these foods are completely free of starches, sugars or grains at every step of the process or, even if they once were, if the ingredients might someday change.

As for diets purporting to be "like SCD" or "based on SCD," they may include foods or supplements that are not permitted on the Specific Carbohydrate Diet and, therefore, could interfere with healing. Our advice is simple: there is only one Specific Carbohydrate Diet, and it is described in the pages of this book.

The progress of science implies not only the accumulation of knowledge, but its organization, its unification, and this involves the periodic invention of new syntheses, coordinating existing knowledge, and of new hypotheses which give us methods of approaching the unknown.

George Sarton
Introduction to the *History of Science*

DEDICATION

This book is dedicated to the memory of
Dr. Sidney Valentine Haas
who first showed me the importance of understanding
the effect of food on the body.

TABLE OF CONTENTS

FOREWORD

Upon discovering *Food and the Gut Reaction*, the first edition of *Breaking the Vicious Cycle: Intestinal Health Through Diet*, I realized that it contained a useful solution for the dietary treatment of many gastrointestinal disorders. By introducing the approach of the "Specific Carbohydrate Diet," it enables patients to thrive on a varied diet that very often reduces symptoms and allows healing of an inflamed intestinal tract. Simply presented, yet sophisticated in its conception, the "Specific Carbohydrate Diet" transcends several oversimplifications to which patients with gastrointestinal problems and their physicians often fall prey.

Several years ago my book, *Seven Weeks to a Settled Stomach* (Simon and Schuster), was published. Since that time, I have earned a reputation as a trouble-shooter for gastrointestinal problems. Patients from many parts of the country have consulted me. Many complain of symptoms consistent with irritable bowel syndrome. Others have been diagnosed formally with classic inflammatory bowel disease. And though some patients have responded well to the usual arsenal of natural digestive aids, intestinal flora replacement, elimination diets, conventional antifungal drugs and antibiotics, still others found no relief.

Food and the Gut Reaction, the first edition of this book, was introduced to me by a colleague and friend, Dr. Leo Galland. He mentioned the book after one of his patients brought the book to his attention. I immediately recognized Elaine Gottschall's book as a potential godsend to my patients. Its value lay in providing a palatable but potent alternative to those dietary approaches commonly in use for management of gastrointestinal problems: the high-fiber diet; the low-fat diet; the low-residue diet; the anti-yeast diet; the gluten-free diet; and other elimination diets.

Based on my experience with patients, I already had reason to question the complex carbohydrate plan as the most
healthy eating program, especially for patients with gastrointestinal complaints. Many gastroenterologists, like most North
American physicians, propound this "low-cholesterol" diet plan. Fat,
it is reasoned, is the bane not only of arteries but also of the intestinal tract: in combination with excess animal protein, so it is said, fat
sets the stage for a host of Western ills from diverticulosis to appen-
dicitis and colon cancer.

Unquestionably, some patients are excellent fiber respon-
ders, but others do poorly with common sources of roughage.
The radical alternative, a meat and salad diet that eliminates
all sugars and starches, is unpalatable and unenforceable for
all but the most dedicated patients. In fact, this strict vegetable
and protein diet, sometimes referred to as the "caveman diet,"
is dangerous for marginally nourished, underweight patients
with Crohn's disease or ulcerative colitis.

One oversimplification Elaine Gottschall's book avoids is
the notion that food allergy is the source of many gastrointestinal complaints. Since dietary manipulation can produce
results, it is, perhaps, natural to assume this. But over-reliance on the
ambiguous results of allergy testing leaves many patients incompletely treated. The more sophisticated belief that it is not individual foods
themselves but the *byproducts* of ingestion of certain foods that cause
intestinal problems is fast replacing the concept of food allergy.

This theory was first set forth by Dr. J.O. Hunter in a landmark *Lancet* article in 1991. Elaine Gottschall's "Specific
Carbohydrate Diet" is an acknowledgement of Hunter's theory.
Another recent *Lancet* article underscores the frequency of intolerances to corn, wheat, milk, potatoes, and rye. This may be the reason
why patients who derive inconsistent benefits from the gluten-free
and lactose-free diets respond so completely to the regimen set forth
in Elaine Gottschall's book. This diet addresses carbohydrate intolerance more broadly than other approaches. The second edition of *Food
and the Gut Reaction, Breaking the Vicious Cycle: Intestinal Health
Through Diet,* should be among the vital resources of every gastroenterologist.

Other corrective strategies amount to a preoccupation with eradicating intestinal pathogens. Those who take this approach believe in the "find a bug, use a drug" philosophy. Elaine Gottschall substitutes the more holistic goal of re-establishing the healthy balance of intestinal flora.

As I began placing patients on the "Specific Carbohydrate Diet," using *Food and the Gut Reaction* as a comprehensive guide, I became impressed with the results. Many patients with Crohn's disease, ulcerative colitis, irritable bowel syndrome and even refractory constipation, found relief although their progress had been stymied previously with elaborate but unsuccessful elimination schemes. The clinical value of the "Specific Carbohydrate Diet" was unquestionable, but interestingly, I began to notice other unanticipated benefits. Patients with muscle aches, stiff joints, and even full-blown arthritis, chronic skin rashes, psoriasis, generalized fatigue and "spaciness" experienced an alleviation of these symptoms. Elaine Gottschall's diet had probably reduced intestinal toxicity.

Unfortunately, the chances of wider acceptance of dietary approaches like this one are small. While many of my innovative, nutritionally-oriented colleagues have availed themselves of *Food and the Gut Reaction* and introduced patients to this approach, most gastroenterologists are, sadly, not even curious. They scarcely acknowledge the role diet can play. For example, a recent Lancet article demonstrating the efficacy of the exclusion diet in the treatment of Crohn's disease has not prompted a single gastroenterologist in my large metropolitan community to administer a facsimile of the successful diet to patients – even when their diseases do not respond to the most skillfully administered drug treatment.

Fortunately, increasing numbers of patients are recognizing the need to break away from total dependency on drugs and symptom-oriented medical care. Many have endured years of suffering, coupled with economic and mental stress, and they are willing to try a wholesome diet, grounded in medical research, which makes sense. The reception given to *Food and the Gut Reaction* (the first edition of this book) by patients has the makings of a true grassroots uprising. Patients, en masse, are willing to try the diet, and many are finding that it works.

Elaine Gottschall is a tireless crusader on behalf of her natural approach to digestive problems. She selflessly gives of her time, love, compassion, attention, and concern to patients and clinicians alike. She has become an energetic cheerleader for many of my patients and has provided invaluable direction when progress has faltered. Her reward is surely the secure knowledge that she has made a difference in the lives of thousands of patients with gastrointestinal disorders.

Ronald L. Hoffman, M.D.
Hoffman Center
40 East 30th St.
New York, New York
10016
June, 1994

Chapter 1

PAST AND PRESENT

In 1951, after many years of clinical experience, Drs. Sidney V. and Merrill P. Haas published a book entitled *Management of Celiac Disease*. Directed to the medical community, the book documented the doctors' experiences in treating and curing hundreds of cases of celiac disease as well as cases of cystic fibrosis of the pancreas.[1] Their approach was dietary, and they used a well-balanced, normal diet that was highly specific as to the types of sugars and starches allowed. When patients followed this Specific Carbohydrate Diet for a minimum of one year, they were then able to return to a normal diet with complete and permanent disappearance of symptoms.

In 1958, we took our eight-year-old daughter to the Drs. Haas. Three years before she had been diagnosed by specialists as having incurable ulcerative colitis, and her condition was deteriorating. The years of treatment with cortisone and sulfonamides, plus innumerable other medical approaches, had been unsuccessful and surgery seemed imminent. The Drs. Haas placed her on the Specific Carbohydrate Diet, and within two years she was free of symptoms. She returned to eating normally after another few years and has remained in excellent health for over twenty years.

Many students, friends, and others whom I have seen in my practice who were suffering from ulcerative colitis, Crohn's disease, celiac disease (not cured by a gluten-free diet), diverticulitis, and various types of chronic diarrhea have tried the Haas Diet and most of them are now free of their respective diseases. Some of the most dramatic and fastest recoveries have occurred in babies and young children with severe constipation and among children who, along with intestinal problems, had serious behavior problems. These included autistic-type hypoactivity as well as hyperactivity, often accompanied by severe and prolonged night terrors. Very often the behavior problems and night terrors cleared within ten days after initiation of the Haas Specific Carbohydrate Diet. It is interesting to note that in June, 1985, the Schizophrenia Association of Great Britain launched a research project to investigate Dr. F. C. Dohan's research concerning a relationship between celiac disease and schizophrenia. The basis for this project is a strict grain-free, milk-free, low sugar diet, closely related to the Specific Carbohydrate Diet.[2,3]

Meanwhile in research laboratories throughout the world, investigators have been studying intestinal problems. Physicians and researchers have found that a special type of synthetic diet (chemical nutrients assembled in the laboratory) called an Elemental Diet shows great promise in the treatment of digestive and intestinal problems of all types. The malabsorption problem seen in cystic fibrosis of the pancreas as well as diarrhea which occurs after cancer chemotherapy have been overcome by the use of the synthetic Elemental Diet.[4,5] When used for patients with Crohn's disease, not only did symptoms disappear but children who had not grown properly for years showed dramatic weight and height gains while on the diet.[6] The level of sodium chloride in the perspiration (the sweat test which measures the severity of the condition) of children with cystic fibrosis of the pancreas decreased dramatically when these children were given the Elemental Diet.[7] Over six hundred scientific publications have appeared in medical journals in the 1970s and early 1980s testifying to the fact that this Elemental Diet is effective in correcting malabsorption and reversing the course of many intestinal disorders.[4] However, since the Elemental Diet is an artificial diet, usually administered via a stomach tube, it cannot be continued indefinitely. When it is discontinued, usually after six to eight weeks, improvement gradually decreases and symptoms usually return.

The common denominator underlying the effectiveness of both the natural Specific Carbohydrate Diet and the synthetic Elemental Diet is the type of carbohydrate which predominates. In the synthetic Elemental Diet, the principal carbohydrate is the single sugar, glucose, which, in biochemical circles, is called a monosaccharide (mono=one; saccharide=sugar) as contrasted with a two-sugar disaccharide such as sucrose (table sugar) or a many-sugar polysaccharide such as starch.

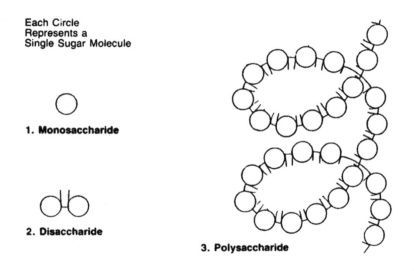

Each Circle
Represents a
Single Sugar Molecule

1. **Monosaccharide**

2. **Disaccharide**

3. **Polysaccharide**

Figure 1   Dietary carbohydrates

In the natural Specific Carbohydrate Diet, the carbohydrates are also predominantly single sugars – those found in fruit, honey, properly-made yogurt, and certain vegetables. The many research reports indicating that the synthetic Elemental Diet is beneficial in intestinal diseases provide support for the Specific Carbohydrate Diet which can be used in the home.

Those who choose to follow the Specific Carbohydrate Diet need not feel deprived. Many of the delicious recipes in this book could easily be part of any gourmet cookbook. The fact that they are so appealing, however, in no way compromises the underlying scientific reasoning: the carbohydrates specified in the recipes are biochemically correct.

The Specific Carbohydrate Diet presented in this book is highly nutritious and well-balanced. It is safe and very likely to be effective in overcoming many lingering and vexing intestinal and digestive problems.

Chapter 2

SCIENTIFIC EVIDENCE RELATING TO DIET

The distressing and debilitating intestinal problems seen today have existed for centuries. The names given the various conditions with the symptoms of diarrhea, excess gas, loss of weight, excess mucus, cramping, blood loss, and severe constipation have changed throughout the years. The methods of diagnosis as well as those of treatment and management have also changed with time. But always, there has been a strong underlying belief that diet is an important factor to consider, not only in determining the causes of the disorders, but also in their treatment and cure.

The medical literature is rich with reports relating the favorable effects of dietary changes on the course of intestinal disease. As far back as 300 A.D., a Roman physician described in detail a diarrhea condition sounding like celiac disease and suggested that fasting, along with the use of the juice of the plantain, a member of the banana family, would cure the disease.[1] In 1745, Prince Charles, the Young Pretender to the throne of England, suffered from ulcerative colitis and was said to have cured himself by adopting a milk-free diet.[2]

During the early 1900s, numerous physicians brought further insight to our understanding of the effect of food on intestinal problems. Dr. Christian Herter, a physician and professor at Columbia University, noted that in every case where children were wasting away with diarrhea and debilitation, proteins were well tolerated, fats were handled moderately well but carbohydrates (sugars and starches) were badly tolerated. He stated that ingestion of some carbohydrates almost invariably caused a relapse or a return of diarrhea after a period of improvement.[3,4] About that time, Dr. Samuel Gee, another world-renowned children's specialist, saw clearly several important facts that continue to be missed by modern researchers. Dr. Gee said that if the patient with intestinal disease could be cured at all, it would have to be by means of diet.[5] He added that milk was the least suitable food during intestinal problems and that highly starchy food (rice, corn, potatoes, grains) were unfit. Dr. Gee stated, "We must never forget that what the patient takes beyond his power to digest does harm." Any food, and particularly carbohydrate, given to a person with intestinal problems should, therefore, be a food that requires little or no digestion so that the digestive process itself will not stand in the way of the absorption of the carbohydrates. Contrary to what some may think, undigested (and, therefore, unabsorbed) carbohydrates are not passing harmlessly through the small intestine and colon and out in the feces but, somehow and somewhere in the digestive tract, are causing problems.

There is much recent evidence to support the hypothesis that the course of several forms of intestinal problems can be favorably changed by manipulating the types of carbohydrates ingested. Cystic fibrosis patients have responded remarkably well to the removal of certain carbohydrates from their diets, especially refined sugar (sucrose) and the milk sugar, lactose, as well as starch.[6-9] Lactose has been implicated over and over again in ulcerative colitis, Crohn's disease, and other types of intestinal disorders referred to as "functional" diarrhea.[10-13] The removal of lactose from the diets of patients with these problems has resulted in remarkable improvement.[14-18]

Crohn's disease research has yielded some dramatic results relating to carbohydrates in the diet. In the 1980s two reports appeared in the medical literature. The first reported the results of Drs. Von Brandes and Lorenz-Meyer of Marburg, West Germany who brought about remissions in twenty patients with Crohn's disease by forbidding foods and beverages containing refined carbohydrates, mainly sucrose and starch.[19] In the second study involving twenty patients with Crohn's disease, dietary changes involving the elimination of specific foods, particularly cereals and dairy products, resulted in sustained remissions. The physicians conducting the research concluded that "dietary manipulation might be an effective long-term therapeutic strategy for Crohn's disease."[20]

A recent medical textbook on the subject of inflammatory bowel disease reported the results of twenty worldwide studies on the eating patterns of patients with ulcerative colitis and Crohn's disease prior to the onset of symptoms and subsequent diagnosis. Two of three studies on the dietary habits of ulcerative colitis patients showed a high consumption of bread and potatoes along with a high intake of refined sugar (sucrose). In one of the studies, a large one comprised of 124 patients, it was concluded that "a dietary factor in ulcerative colitis cannot be dismissed, especially in relation to bread."[26] In this same textbook, the results of seventeen studies dealing with Crohn's disease were reported, and all studies found sucrose intake to be, higher in Crohn's patients than in people without Crohn's disease. The author of the report stated:

> The consistency of this finding is remarkable considering the variety of countries and methods used to carry out the studies.

Among the patients in the seventeen studies reported, it was found that sucrose intake varied from between 20% to 220% more in Crohn's patients than in people who did not develop Crohn's disease.

In concluding, Dr. Heaton, author of the report, stated:

> The connection between Crohn's disease and a sugar-rich diet is proved beyond reasonable doubt. Apart from smoking, this is the strongest clue to an environmental etiology of the disease.[26]

Dr. Claude Morin of Hospital Sainte-Justine, Quebec, reported his results in treating four children who were suffering from long-standing Crohn's disease.

When Dr. Morin administered, via a stomach tube, a synthetic elemental diet containing the monosaccharide glucose (a single sugar) as the main carbohydrate source, the children showed remarkable gains in both height and weight as well as remission of their symptoms.[21] Unlike sucrose, lactose, and starch, *glucose requires no digestion* and is, therefore, more likely to be absorbed by the cells of the small intestine. This "predigested" sugar can easily pass through the intestinal absorptive cells, enter the bloodstream and nourish the body. Glucose in the synthetic elemental diet as well as glucose found in fruits and honey is not beyond the power of those with disturbed digestive systems to absorb.

Dr. Jan Van Eys of the University of Texas Cancer Center reaffirmed this principle by stating:

> The gastrointestinal mucosa (surface) of children is especially prone to damage from diarrhea and, as a result, disaccharide intolerance. The development of disaccharide-deficient formulae and of elemental diets gave a means by which physicians could allow patients to recover without drastic measures.[22]

Dr. Van Eys did not elaborate on the conditions that lead to the inability to digest double sugars (disaccharides) nor did he state how diarrhea is related to the problem of disaccharide digestion. More recently, however, Dr. J. Ranier Poley of Eastern Virginia Medical School has shown a link between diarrhea and the inability to digest starch and disaccharide sugars.[23] By microscopically examining the intestinal surface of patients with various forms of diarrhea, Dr. Poley found that most patients have lost the ability to digest disaccharides because of excessive mucus production by intestinal cells. An abnormally thick layer of surface mucus appears to be preventing contact between the disaccharides and the digestive enzymes of the absorptive cells. Sugars that need digestion cannot be processed and, therefore, will not be absorbed to provide nourishment for the individual. Dr. Poley has shown this phenomenon to take place in those suffering with celiac disease (gluten-sensitive enteropathy), soy-protein intolerance, intolerance to cow's milk protein, intractable diarrhea of infancy, chronic diarrhea in children, parasitic infections of the intestine (Giardia), cystic fibrosis of the pancreas, and Crohn's disease.[23] Reasons for the production of excessive mucus will be discussed in greater detail in the next chapter dealing with intestinal microbes.

Carbohydrates (sugars and starches) will be discussed in Chapter 5 in order to understand how some are more likely than others to escape digestion and, therefore, absorption. It will become clear that when this occurs, they remain in the intestinal tract and are utilized by the microbial world of the intestine which depends on this available carbohydrate for

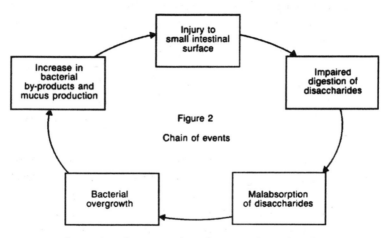

Figure 2

Chain of events

the energy the microbes need to live and multiply.[24] Yeast and bacteria change the carbohydrates in ways that can injure the intestine which may respond to these microbial by-products by secreting excessive mucus. A chain of events (Figure 2) is then established.

At present, it is difficult to pinpoint the first step that triggers the cycle involving dietary carbohydrates and intestinal microbial growth. As far back as 1922, in a speech to the medical community entitled, "Faulty Food in Relation to Gastrointestinal Disorders," Dr. Robert McCarrison warned his colleagues that intestinal diseases were increasing. He asked them to remember that microbes, often blamed for intestinal disease, are dependent upon the conditions of life, especially nutrition, which "frequently prepare the soil of the body for

the growth of these microorganisms."[25] It is reasonable to
believe that undigested, unabsorbed carbohydrates remaining
in the intestine can serve as "the soil of the body" which
encourages the growth of microorganisms involved in intestinal disorders.

In various conditions, a poorly-functioning intestine can
be easily overwhelmed by the ingestion of carbohydrates
which requires numerous digestive processes. The result is an
environment that supports overgrowth of intestinal yeast and bacteria thus either initiating the chain of events or perpetuating it.

The purpose of the Specific Carbohydrate Diet is to
deprive the microbial world of the intestine of the food it
needs to overpopulate. By using a diet which contains
predominantly "predigested" carbohydrates, the individual
with an intestinal problem can be maximally nourished
without over-stimulation of the intestinal microbial
population.

Chapter 3

INTESTINAL MICROBES: THE UNSEEN WORLD

The two most hazardous things an astronaut takes into his capsule on extended flight are his brain and his intestinal flora.† (Bengson)[1]

A man is only what his microbes make him. (Ropeloff)[2]

It is generally accepted among physicians and researchers that during intestinal upsets and chronic intestinal disease, the normal, harmonious state of balance between intestinal microbes living in our gastrointestinal tract is lost. It is important, therefore, that we have some understanding of the inhabitants of our unseen world.

Before birth, the human intestine is free of microbes.[3,4] From the moment of birth, however, a massive invasion of the gastrointestinal tract takes place and it soon becomes populated with various types of microbes depending on the type of milk ingested as well as other environmental factors. Some of the microbial growth develops from contact with the mother's skin; some originates from the air. If the infant is breastfed, more than 99% of all microbes in the intestine are of one type.[3] As other foods are introduced, the baby develops a wide variety of bacteria.

Studies have revealed that eventually more than four hundred bacterial species live together in the human colon.[52] The stomach and most of the small intestine do not normally har-

† *intestinal flora – the various bacterial and other microscopic forms of life in the intestinal contents.*

bor more than a sparse population of microbial flora. However, the number of microbes normally increases at the lowest part of the small intestine, the ileum, because of its close proximity to the microbial-rich colon.[5]

In the healthy intestinal tract, intestinal microbes appear to live in a state of balance; an overabundance of one type

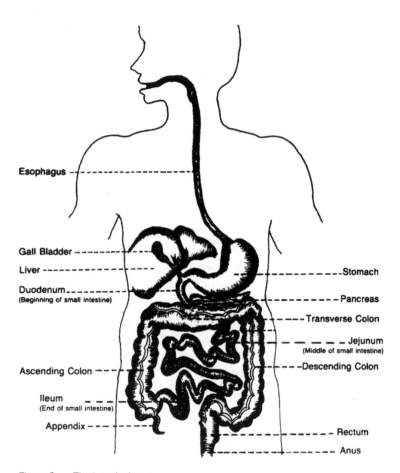

Figure 3   The intestinal tract

seems to be inhibited by the activities of other types. This competition between microbes prevents any one type from overwhelming the body with its waste products or toxins. Another important protective factor which works to maintain the sparse bacterial population of the stomach and upper small intestine is the high acidity of the stomach's hydrochloric acid in which microbes cannot usually survive. In addition, normal peristalsis (waves of involuntary muscular contractions) sweeps many microbes out of the intestine to be lost in the feces, thereby decreasing their numbers.

However, bacterial overgrowth in the stomach and small intestine can and does occur for various reasons among which are:

(1) Interference with the high acidity of the stomach through the continual use of antacids;

(2) A decrease in the acidity of the stomach such as occurs in the aging process [6];

(3) Malnutrition or a diet of poor quality, and the resulting weakening of the body's immune system[7,8];

(4) Antibiotic therapy which can cause a wide range of microbial changes. A microbe commonly residing in the intestine without harmful effects may undergo a wide range of changes as a result of antibiotic therapy.[9]

Once the normal equilibrium of the colon is disturbed for any reason, its microbes can migrate into the small intestine and stomach hampering digestion, competing for nutrients, and overloading the intestinal tract with their waste products.[3] Quite early in bacterial overgrowth of the small intestine, the normal absorption of vitamin B12 is disturbed. There is considerable evidence that B12 is poorly absorbed when microbes multiplying within the small intestine prevent uptake by the ileum.[12,13]

There has been a long history indicating that bacteria and yeast are involved in intestinal disease. As far back as 1904, an examination of the stools of children who were suffering with what appeared to be celiac disease, revealed abnormally large numbers of fermentative (carbohydrate "eaters") and putrefactive (protein "eaters") bacteria which were, undoubtedly, contributing to the disease process. The physicians making this observation proposed that although the normal intestine controlled the growth of bacteria, in "celiac-type" cases some intestinal abnormality prevented the normal regulatory control.[14]

Early researchers working on ulcerative colitis believed this disorder to be caused by bacteria. From 1906 to 1924, numerous researchers isolated certain types of bacteria, injected either the bacteria or the bacterial toxins into laboratory animals, and claimed that the injections produced ulcerative colitis in the animals.[15-18] In 1932, when Dr. B.B. Crohn spoke about a "new" intestinal disorder which he called regional ileitis (now known as Crohn's disease), some physicians attending his lecture stated that this new disease entity might be due to microorganisms.[19]

From the 1920s until the present, the role of microbes and the products they produce continues to be investigated in an effort to find the cause of the various forms of inflammatory bowel disease.[20-26] Often there has been very convincing evidence that particular bacteria could initiate a certain type of intestinal disease but, eventually, the work has been dismissed because of insufficient proof. Some of the difficulties which these investigators experienced in trying to pinpoint the "culprit" microbes were undoubtedly due to the ever-changing conditions of the microbial world of the intestine, to variability in the strains of intestinal microbes, or to the lack of precise laboratory techniques of identification.

During these early years of investigation, Dr. Ilya Metchnikoff proposed that bacteria in the intestine were producing toxins which were then absorbed into the bloodstream. These toxins, Metchnikoff stated, were the cause of many human afflictions, and he named the process by which harmful microbes in the intestine cause disease, "autointoxication."[27] Unlike investigators who unsuccessfully attempted to find the precise microorganisms involved in the various types of intestinal disorders, Metchnikoff approached the problem quite differently. He maintained, as many others have done, that if the intestinal environment can be kept in a healthy state, harmful microbes will no longer be a threat.[30]

He advocated the widespread use of acidified (fermented) milk, similar to yogurt, and proposed that the beneficial bacteria used in producing the fermented milk, and still remaining therein, would enter the intestinal tract and prevent other bacteria in the intestine from forming harmful toxins. While Metchnikoff's proposal has not been universally adopted, his ideas are acknowledged by outstanding gastroenterologists and researchers. In 1964, Dr. Donaldson stated in a lengthy article about the role of bacteria in intestinal disease, "in certain respects the concept of autointoxication offered by Metchnikoff must now receive serious reconsideration."[12]

Investigators continue to be fascinated by Metchnikoff's proposals and to study the potential benefits of acidified milk. Modern researchers are asking: Do the bacteria used to ferment the milk actually take up residence in the intestine and, if so, for how long? Which of the "yogurt-type" bacteria used to acidify milk will counteract toxins produced by other intestinal microbes?[28] Is the bacteria used to acidify the milk or the acidified (fermented) milk itself the beneficial factor?[29]

In the 1980s an increasing number of reports have been published stating that intestinal bacterial toxins appear to be injuring intestinal cells and, as a result, causing a variety of diarrheal diseases. Some of the bacteria producing these toxins have not, in the past, been considered to be disease-causing types.[7] Although there is still insufficient evidence to link a specific microbe to each of the chronic intestinal disorders, it is generally agreed that intestinal microbes are not innocent bystanders.

A simple approach to minimizing the undesirable activities of intestinal microbes would seem to be through the use of antibiotics. This approach is often tried but, unfortunately, in most chronic intestinal disorders, it has limitations.[31-48]

We are faced, then, with intestinal disorders which involve microbial populations which have been altered in number, in kind, or both. The normal contractions (peristalsis) of the intestinal muscles are not able to remove them; they appear to be tenacious. Indeed, there is evidence that intestinal microbes will not cause disease unless they develop methods of adhering to the gut wall.[49,50] Antibiotic therapy is of limited usefulness while other drugs of the cortisone and sulfa families have side-effects if continued too long.

A sensible and harmless form of warfare on the aberrant population of intestinal microbes is to manipulate their energy (food) supply through diet. Most intestinal microbes require carbohydrates for energy,[51] and the Specific Carbohydrate Diet severely limits the availability of carbohydrates. By depriving intestinal microbes of their energy source, their numbers gradually decrease along with the products they produce.

Chapter 4

BREAKING THE VICIOUS CYCLE

Of all dietary components, carbohydrate has the major influence over intestinal microbes. Through a process of fermentation of available carbohydrates remaining in the intestinal tract, microbes obtain energy for continued maintenance and growth.[1]

The fermentation process by which intestinal microbes consume dietary carbohydrates is diagrammed below:

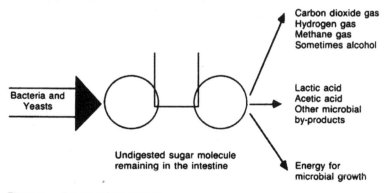

Figure 4   Intestinal fermentation

Fermentation is encouraged when the diet contains carbohydrates which remain in the intestinal tract rather than being absorbed into the bloodstream.[2] Unabsorbed carbohydrates constitute the most important source of gas in the intestine. For example, the lactose contained in one ounce of milk, if undigested and unabsorbed, will produce about 50 ml of gas in the intestine of normal people. But under abnormal conditions when intestinal microbes have moved into the small intestine, the hydrogen gas production may be increased over one hundred-fold.

The presence of undigested and unabsorbed carbohydrates within the small intestine can encourage microbes from the colon to take up residence in the small intestine and to continue to multiply. This, in turn, may lead to the formation of products, in addition to gas, which injure the small intestine. Examples are lactic, acetic, and other acids (Fig. 4) which are short-chain organic acids resulting from the fermentative process. In addition to the damage to the intestine, there is a growing body of scientific evidence that lactic acid formed from fermentation in the intestine causes abnormal brain function and behavior,[3,4,5] which could account for the behavioral problems which often accompany intestinal disorders. This would also explain the dramatic improvements in behavior noted in Chapter 1: the formation of large amounts of lactic acid resulting from the fermentation of unabsorbed carbohydrates is prevented by following the Specific Carbohydrate Diet.

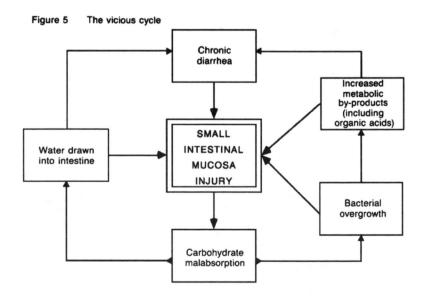

Figure 5   The vicious cycle

The production of large amounts of short-chain organic acids by bacterial fermentation in the intestine may ultimately prove to be an important clue in discovering the cause of some forms of inflammatory bowel disease.

A recently published paper in Science entitled "Grain Feeding and the Dissemination of Acid-Resistant Escherichia coli from Cattle" casts a new perspective on the effect of these organic acids in changing bacterial characteristics.[11] Since the early 1980s medical research has shown that some forms of ulcerative colitis appear to be caused by a commonly-found intestinal bacterium, Escherichia coli, which, as a result of a change in its characteristics (a mutation), has developed the ability to produce disease.[12-14] Although there are numerous reasons as to why harmless forms of bacteria might change their characteristics through genetic mutation, the question could be asked: Is the fermentation of undigested, unabsorbed starch by intestinal bacteria in the human colon causing an acidic environment which could cause harmless bacteria to change to harmful forms?

Once bacteria multiply within the small intestine, the chain of events diagrammed in Figure 5 develops into a vicious cycle characterized by an increase in the production of gas, acids and other products of fermentation which perpetuate the malabsorption problem and prolong the intestinal disorder.[6]

Bacterial growth in the small intestine appears to destroy the enzymes on the intestinal cell surface preventing carbohydrate digestion and absorption and making carbohydrates available for further fermentation.[7] It is at this point that production of excessive mucus may be triggered as a self-defense mechanism whereby the intestinal tract attempts to "lubricate" itself against the mechanical and chemical injury caused by the microbial toxins, acids, and the presence of incompletely digested and unabsorbed carbohydrates.

The Specific Carbohydrate Diet presents a method for breaking the cycle by maximally nourishing the individual and minimally nourishing the intestinal microbes. By this method, undesirable stresses on the intestine decrease. The diet is based on the principle that specifically selected carbo-hydrates, requiring minimal digestive processes (as will be discussed in Chapter 5) are absorbed and leave virtually none to be used for furthering microbial growth in the intestine. As the microbial population decreases due to lack of food, its harmful by-products also decrease, freeing the intestinal sur-face of injurious substances. No longer needing protection, the mucus-producing cells stop producing excessive mucus, and carbohydrate digestion is improved. Malabsorption is replaced by absorption. As the individual absorbs energy and nutrients, all the cells of the body are properly nourished, including the cells of the immune system, which then can assist in overcoming the microbial invasion. The practical Specific Carbohydrate Diet aims for the same goals as the clinical synthetic Elemental Diet: the reduction and change of bacterial growth and the maintenance of the optimum nutri-tional state of the patient.[9,10]

Chapter 5

CARBOHYDRATE DIGESTION

Digestion is the great secret of life. (Go and Summerskill)[1]

What the patient takes beyond his ability to digest does harm. (Gee)[2]

While the underlying causes of the various intestinal disorders cannot be stated with certainty, faulty digestion and malabsorption of dietary carbohydrates may be, in large part, responsible for these disorders. (Carbohydrate refers to starch and disaccharide sugar molecules; both require digestion before absorption.) As we have seen in previous chapters, this can lead to more serious malabsorption of all nutrients due to injury to the intestinal surface. The Specific Carbohydrate Diet most often corrects malabsorption allowing nutrients to enter the bloodstream and be made available to the cells of the body, thereby strengthening the immune system's ability to fight. Further debilitation is prevented, weight can return to normal and, ultimately, there is a return to health.

Malabsorption is the inability of the cells of the body to obtain nutrients from foods eaten. As a result, the caloric energy, vitamins, and minerals are lost as all parts of the body are deprived of the proper nourishment. There are many places in the gastrointestinal tract where problems could lead to malabsorption: (1) if food travels too rapidly through the intestinal tract (as happens most often when diarrhea is present), there is insufficient time for large food molecules such as starch, fat and protein to be broken down by various enzymes and, consequently, their absorption into the bloodstream is seriously impaired; (2) if a poorly functioning pancreas does not deliver sufficient digestive enzymes to the small intestine to break down large molecules of protein, fat, and starch, absorption of these nutrients will not take place.

However, a large number of research reports point to a later step in digestion as the site leading to malabsorption in many intestinal disorders.[4,5,8-14,16,18] This last step in the digestive process occurs at the microvilli of the cell membranes of the intestinal absorptive cell.

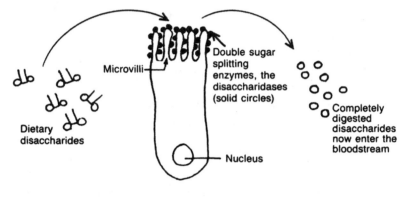

Figure 6   Tall, healthy, mature intestinal absorptive cell

The membranes of cells lining the intestinal tract serve as more than a passive barrier between the contents of the digestive tract and the bloodstream. When the digestive system is functioning normally, the membranes of these "gatekeeper" cells *actively* participate in the last step of digestion as well as aiding in the transport of nutrients into the bloodstream.

The last step in carbohydrate digestion takes place at the minute projections called microvilli (Fig. 6). Only those carbohydrates which have been properly processed by the enzymes embedded in the microvilli can cross over the barrier and enter the bloodstream.[3] This is where the milk sugar, lactose, and sucrose are split apart (digested). This is also the site of the last step in the digestion of starch from foods such

Figure 7   Digestion of dietary carbohydrates

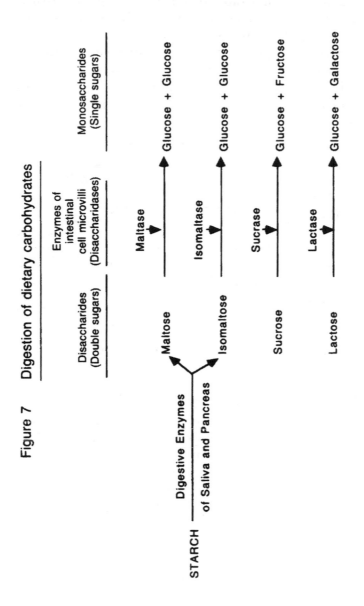

as grains and potatoes. Figure 7 summarizes the steps involved in carbohydrate digestion in the gastrointestinal tract and lists the microvilli enzymes which carry out the last step of the digestive process.

The structure of the intestinal surface is dramatically altered during intestinal disease[4] and, as a result, digestive activity is seriously inhibited. This makes the last step in the digestion of these carbohydrates difficult, if not impossible[4, 12,15] (Fig. 8)

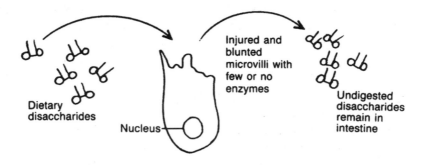

Injured and blunted microvilli with few or no enzymes

Dietary disaccharides

Nucleus

Undigested disaccharides remain in intestine

Figure 8   Flattened, injured, immature absorptive cell

The location of the sugar-splitting enzymes, the disaccharidases, in the membranes of the intestinal cells makes them very vulnerable to damage from many sources. A vitamin deficiency of folic acid,[29] for example, and/or of B12 can prevent proper development of the microvilli which carry the disaccharidases. An abnormally thick layer of mucus produced by the intestinal cells can prevent contact between the microvilli enzymes and the disaccharides lactose, sucrose, maltose and isomaltose.[4] In addition, irritating or toxic substances produced by yeast, bacteria, or parasites which have invaded the small intestinal tract can cause damage to the intestinal cell membranes, destroying their enzymes.[13]

Conditions involving the small intestine that are frequently associated with deficiencies of lactase and other disaccharidases are celiac disease, malnutrition, tropical sprue, cholera, gastroenteritis, infant diarrhea from any cause, pellagra, irritable colon, post-gastrectomy (removal of part of stomach),[14] soy protein intolerance, intolerance to cow's milk protein, intractable diarrhea of infancy, parasitic infections of the intestine, cystic fibrosis, and Crohn's disease.[4,5,8-14,16,18] In addition, lactase deficiency in ulcerative colitis is well documented as was noted in Chapter 2.

The first enzyme to suffer damage is usually lactase, but often there is a combination of enzyme loss involving sucrase, isomaltase, and, less often, maltase.[14] The enzyme, lactase, is depressed earlier than the other disaccharide-splitting enzymes in intestinal disturbances such as celiac disease (and other conditions where diarrhea is present) and is the last of the microvilli enzymes to return to normal after intestinal disease has subsided. In fact, lactase may be permanently depressed after severe malnutrition and tropical diarrhea (sprue) and a deficiency of lactase may be the sole legacy of some previous disorders.[14]

It is difficult to prove the absence of disaccharidase activity by present medical techniques. A biopsy sample of the small intestine during intestinal disease may show that enzyme activity of disaccharidases is normal. However, upon feeding lactose, sucrose, and starch, cramping, diarrhea, and vomiting will follow. This apparent contradiction could be due to a lack of contact between the enzymes and sugars caused by the mucus barrier referred to in Chapters 2 and 3.

When a biopsy sample *does* indicate that there is a deficiency of disaccharidase enzyme activity, the reason could be a primary genetic problem or a secondary problem caused by a direct injury to the intestinal cell surface with loss of the microvilli and a flattening of the cell itself. Among those factors which lead to injuries of the intestinal surface are malnutrition and irritation caused by substances produced by microbial growth.[15,16]

The sugars then remain undigested in the small intestine.[4,17] Their presence in the lumen (interior space) of the intestine causes a reversal of the normal nutritional process. Instead of nutrients flowing from the intestinal space into the bloodstream, water is drawn into the intestinal lumen (Fig. 5). The water, carrying nutrients, is lost in abnormal intestinal function (diarrhea) and the cells of the body are deprived of energy, minerals, and vitamins. Most seriously, the sugars remaining in the intestinal lumen provide energy for further fermentation and growth of intestinal microbes.

The increasing levels of irritating substances given off by the growing microbial population cause intestinal cells to defend themselves. Mucus-producing cells (goblet cells) which are normally present in the intestine secrete their product to cover and protect the naked free surface of the intestinal absorptive cells. The small intestine responds to a disruption of the normal balance by producing more goblet cells which increases the secretion of intestinal mucus. As the integrity of the small intestine is further threatened by the microbial invasion and by the products it produces, a thick mucus barrier forms for self defense. The enzymes embedded within the absorptive cell membranes cannot do the job for which they are designed: to make contact with and split certain sugars in the diet.[4]

If the goblet cells become exhausted (and there is a limit to their valiant efforts to defend the absorptive lining against irritation), the "naked" intestinal surface is subject to further ravaging. It is very possible that, at this stage, ulceration of the intestinal surface, as seen in ulcerative colitis, can occur. This might also explain how certain proteins such as gluten can inappropriately enter the interior of the absorptive cells and destroy them.

Sometimes, but not often, even the absorption of single sugars is disturbed because of severe injury to the absorptive cells, but this extreme condition is usually diagnosed by routine hospital tests.[18] Sometimes, the invasion of microbes into the small intestine is so pervasive that yeast, for example, will be found in the esophagus.[19] When it is suspected that yeast invasion is widespread (the oral infection, thrush, would be an indicator) it is wise to cut back on honey ingestion at the beginning of the dietary regimen (amount of honey in recipes should be decreased by at least 75%). The amount of honey may be increased as the condition improves.

The indigestibility of starch by even healthy people is only recently receiving attention (see descriptions of starches following). Some starchy foods which were assumed to be digested completely are, in fact, incompletely digested by most people.[20,21] In those people with intestinal disorders, the digestibility of starch is even further affected. Because the breakdown of starch eventually results in the formation of the disaccharides, maltose and isomaltose, most starches must be avoided unless they are specified as permissible in Chapter 10.

Some foods in the Specific Carbohydrate Diet contain starches which have been shown to be tolerated. These are the starches of the legume family: dried beans, lentils and split peas (no chick peas, soybeans or bean sprouts). The legumes which are permitted must, however, be soaked for at least 10-12 hours prior to cooking and the water discarded since they contain other sugars which are indigestible but which can be removed by soaking.[22] The legumes may be introduced in small amounts at about the third month of the diet. The starches in all grains, corn, and potatoes must be strictly avoided. Corn syrup is also excluded since it contains a mixture of "short-chain" starches.[23,24]

Carbohydrates Found in Foods

1. Single Sugars (monosaccharides)
These sugars require no further splitting in order to be transported from the intestine into the bloodstream. They are glucose, fructose, and galactose. Glucose and fructose are found in honey, fruits, and some vegetables. Galactose is found in lactose-hydrolyzed milk (LHM) and in yogurt.

2. Double Sugars (disaccharides)
These sugars require splitting by intestinal cell enzymes. There are four main disaccharides: lactose, sucrose, maltose, and isomaltose.

Lactose is found in fluid milk, dried milk powder, commercial yogurt, homemade yogurt which has not been fermented for twenty-four hours, processed cheeses, cottage cheese, cream cheese, ice cream, some sour creams, whey (70% lactose by weight), and many products which have added milk solids or whey. Many drugs and vitamin and mineral supplements have added lactose.

Sucrose is table sugar and is found in processed foods such as gelatin desserts, ketchup, cereals, many canned foods and some frozen preparations (see Appendix). There is a small amount of sucrose (about 1%-3%) in some pasteurized honey but it has been shown to be tolerated by those on the Specific Carbohydrate Diet. Unpasteurized honey contains virtually no sucrose since an enzyme in the honey splits whatever sucrose may be present. Some fruits and nuts contain small amounts of sucrose but they may be used and have been included in Chapter 10. As fruits ripen, some of the sucrose they may contain is split by enzymes within the fruit.

Maltose and **Isomaltose** are found in sources such as corn syrup, malted milk, and candies. However, most of the maltose and isomaltose which is presented to the intestinal cells for digestion comes from dietary starches. Starches are long chains of glucose molecules (Fig. 9) which are digested, in part, by enzymes from the pancreas and saliva and are left as the disaccharides, maltose and isomaltose, to be split by microvilli enzymes of intestinal cells.

3. Starch (polysaccharides)

Starch can be of two types called amylose and amylopectin. Most vegetables contain both types in various proportions. For example, some kinds of rice contain small amounts of amylopectin starch and large amounts of amylose starch. Other types of rice contain only amylopectin starch.[25] Like rice, some genetic strains of corn contain a very highly branched amylopectin type of starch. Sweet potatoes or yams also contain only amylopectin starch. It appears that genetic breeding which attempts to change the protein content of certain crops also affects the types of starch formed by the plant.[25] The varying proportions of different kinds of starch might affect the ability of the intestine to completely digest them. Or, the proteins of certain plants may prevent the starch from being completely split.[27] (It is interesting to note that one group of researchers has found that some intestinal bacteria are made more virulent by the presence of undigested cornstarch in the intestine.[26])

Vegetables that contain more amylose than amylopectin starch are simpler to digest, because the glucose units which make up all starch molecules are arranged in a linear fashion in amylose starch and are readily exposed to digestive enzymes from saliva and the pancreas (Fig. 9). The links holding the glucose units in these linear arrays are split until

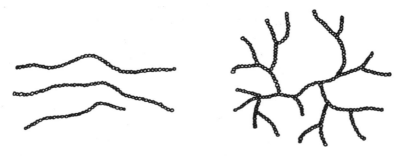

AMYLOSE   AMYLOPECTIN

Each small circle in the above diagrams represents a glucose molecule.

Figure 9   Starches

the chains are reduced to only two chemically linked glucose molecules called maltose. By comparison, amylopectin molecules contain glucose units which form branches (Figs. 9 and 10). When the amylopectin molecules have been partially digested by pancreatic enzymes, the fragments remaining for the last step in digestion by microvilli enzymes are both maltose and isomaltose.

Recently, Dr. Gunja-Smith and associates proposed that the amylopectin starch molecule is even more highly branched than was thought originally.[28]

According to Dr. Gunja-Smith's diagram, the interior branches appear less exposed than the exterior branches. It is, therefore, possible that pancreatic digestive enzymes can not reach the interior links and that parts of the amylopectin starch molecules escape digestion, remain in the intestine, and increase microbial fermention.

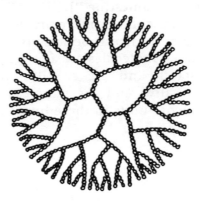

Figure 10   Revised diagram of amylopectin starch

At present, very limited information is available as to the amounts of amylopectin and amylose starch present in the many kinds of grains and other starchy foods.

Fiber: Fruits, vegetables, nuts, and grains contain various components, termed fiber, which are indigestible by the enzymes of the digestive tract. Fiber from fruits, nuts, vegetables, including dried legumes, is allowed on the Specific Carbohydrate Diet but all other fiber from grains, including bran, is not permitted.

Chapter 6

The Celiac Story

The last time anyone counted, there were 15,000 named diseases of man, and cures for 5,000 of them. Yet it remains the dream of every young doctor to discover a new disease. That is the fastest and surest way to gain prominence within the medical profession. Practically speaking, it is much better to discover a new disease than to find a cure for an old one; your cure will be tested, disputed and argued over for years, while a new disease is readily and rapidly accepted. (Michael Crichton)[1]

Celiac disease appears to have always existed. Because its numerous symptoms mimic those of several other conditions and because an obvious cause has been elusive throughout the years, its recognition as a distinct disorder and one which physicians could readily diagnose has been fraught with disagreement.

One of the first descriptions of this disorder was given in the early years of the Roman empire by the physician, Aretaeus, who refers to "Coeliac disease" as a chronic diarrhea condition consisting of undigested food, lasting an extended period, and a debilitation of the whole body.[2]

Aretaeus described the diarrhea as being light in color, offensive in odor and accompanied by flatulence. Additionally, the patient is described as "emaciated and atrophied, pale, feeble, incapable of performing any of his accustomed works."

In 1855, Dr. Gull, writing in Guy's Hospital Reports,[3] outlined the symptoms found in a 13 year-old boy that clearly suggest celiac disease as we understand it today: enlarged abdomen, frequent and voluminous stools of a dull, chalky color.

A few years later, in 1888, Dr. Samuel Gee laid the foundation for not only describing the condition, but also establishing criteria for diagnosis. Additionally, he established guidelines for successfully treating the condition with a dietary approach. In Samuel Gee's classic report, "On the Coeliac Affection," he wrote:

> There is a kind of chronic indigestion which is met with in persons of all ages, yet is especially apt to affect children between one and five years old. Signs of the disease are yielded by the faeces; being loose, not formed, but not watery; more bulky than the food taken would seem to account for; pale in colour, as if devoid of bile, yeasty, frothy, an appearance due to fermentation; stench often very great, the food having undergone putrefaction rather than concoction. The causes of the disease are obscure. Children who suffer from it are not all weak in constitution. Errors in diet may perhaps be a cause, but what error?[4]

Despite the meagerness of Gee's information about celiac disease, he saw clearly several important facts that escaped many later investigations:

(1) If the patient can be cured at all, it must be by means of diet and that cow's milk is the least suited kind of food, that highly starchy food, rice, sago, corn-flour, are unfit.

(2) We must never forget that what the patient takes beyond his power of digestion does harm. (Gee implied that unfit foods played more than a negative role and actually produced a pathologic condition in the digestive tract.)

For many years there were numerous reports on the cause as well as the treatment for what appeared to be celiac. While these inconsistent and inconclusive reports appeared in Europe, there was much less interest in North America. Shortly after the turn of the century, however, Drs. L. Emmett

Holt Sr., Director of Children's Medicine at Bellevue Hospital and Christian Herter of Columbia University worked together for over 7 years on the clinical as well as the theoretical aspects of this disorder. Their conclusions, published in 1908 entitled *On Infantilism from Chronic Intestinal Infection*, included the following main points:

(1) There is a pathological state of childhood marked by a striking retardation in growth of the skeleton, the muscles, and the various organs that is associated with a chronic intestinal infection characterized by the overgrowth and persistence of bacterial flora belonging normally to the nursling period.

(2) The chief manifestations of this intestinal infantilism are arrest in the development of the body but maintenance of good mental powers and a fair development of the brain; marked abdominal distention; a slight or moderate or considerable degree of simple anemia; the rapid onset of physical and mental fatigue; irregularities of intestinal digestion resulting in frequent diarrheal seizures.[5]

Drs. Holt and Herter continued in their monograph to describe the dominant bacteria found in the stools as well as some of the by-products of intestinal fermentation and putrefaction. They noted that fat appeared in the stool and attributed this to impaired fat absorption. Also, note was made of increased mucus in the stool along with evidence of abnormal shedding of intestinal cells. They continued to stress that two leading features of this intestinal infantilism must be further investigated: (1) the retardation of growth; (2) the chronic intoxication. They commented that retardation in growth could be attributed to malabsorption of nutrients and the malabsorption could probably be due to a chronic inflammation located in the ileum and colon associated with the presence of .abnormal forms of bacteria. The chronic intoxication, they were certain, resulted from the action of products of bacterial origin with the toxins having as their main target the nervous system and muscles.

They concluded their treatise by stating:

> Temporary relapses are very common in the course of this disease, even when great care is being taken to prevent them. The most frequent cause of such relapses is the attempt to encourage growth by the use of increased amounts of carbohydrates.

Although Herter's conclusions failed to gain acceptance, his observations were so perceptive that further researchers "stood on his shoulders" in pursuing the most effective dietary treatment. He saw that in every case proteins were very well handled, fats were handled moderately well, while carbohydrates were badly tolerated, almost invariably causing relapse or a return of diarrhea after a period of improvement. He said, "It has been already mentioned that the carbohydrates are the obvious and fruitful cause of derangements of digestion that are clinically determinable, especially diarrhea and flatulence."

Meanwhile, the interest shown by Drs. Holt and Herter had been transmitted to Dr. Holt's two younger assistants at the Vanderbilt Clinic, Dr. John Howland and Dr. Sidney V. Haas. In 1921, Howland, in his presidential address before the American Pediatric Society, read a paper on "Prolonged Intolerance to Carbohydrates."[6] Although Howland did not use the term celiac disease (the condition was still known by a great variety of names) he described his cases vividly:

> There are loose stools from time to time with loss of weight. The condition improves between the attacks somewhat, but sooner or later a relapse occurs and there is a renewed loss of weight. The relapses are increasingly severe. Eventually, there is a condition of marked malnutrition in a peevish, fretful, but often precocious child. The abdomen is distended, at first intermittently, and then almost constantly. The stools are never normal. Even between attacks of diarrhea they are large, light gray in color, often frothy, and usually very foul... Growth suffers in proportion to the length of time that the symptoms persist, and many children are greatly below the average in

height. From clinical experience, it has been found that of all the elements of food, carbohydrates is the one which must be excluded rigorously; that with this greatly reduced, the protein and fat are almost always well digested even though the absorption of fat may not be as satisfactory as in health.

Dr. Howland warned that after initial improvement occurs with the elimination of carbohydrates, the stage where carbohydrates are added is the most difficult. He explained that although the initial phase may be time consuming, "these patients well repay the efforts expended on them. They do not remain semi-invalids, many become vigorous and strong, some even with no trace of dietary idiosyncrasies... Halfway measures are quite unavailing and cause only loss of time." Other doctors confirmed Howland's treatment as achieving greater success than any previous one, but the need for some tolerable carbohydrate in the celiac diet remained.

Despite the remarkable success of Dr. Howland's treatment with emphasis on carbohydrate restriction, other doctors, distracted by the occurrence of fatty stools, continued to believe that dietary fats were at fault. But although there was some confusion resulting from this belief, there was a steadily increasing recognition of the primary role of disordered carbohydrate metabolism and digestion in causing celiac disease.

Dr. Sidney Valentine Haas, working with Dr. Howland, was in full agreement with Dr. Howland's work but was interested in learning if some form of carbohydrate could be added to the diet to hasten recovery and provide a more varied and nutritious diet. He had noted reports throughout the years whereby children with severe diarrhea had done very well on banana flour (made of 70 percent ripe banana) and plantain meal. It was at the Home for Hebrew Infants that Dr. Haas first experimented with banana feeding.[7] One of his patients was an infant who had difficulty in eating. The baby refused all food. Dr. Haas offered the baby a banana. At that time, banana was considered completely indigestible by a sick child. Everybody was horrified at the idea of feeding it to an infant—everybody that is, except the infant, who not only took it but asked for more. He was given more and thus Dr. Haas discovered the banana could be well tolerated.

He then decided to experiment with the banana, as the sought-after carbohydrate source, in the dietary treatment for celiac. He soon discovered that celiacs could tolerate this carbohydrate and, more than that, the banana could be fed in large quantities with beneficial effect. He further experimented with carbohydrate-containing fruits and some vegetables and found that they, too, could be tolerated and the celiac could regain health on a far more varied diet than just protein and fat.

During the next few years, Dr. Haas treated over 600 cases of celiac disease with his Specific Carbohydrate Diet maintaining his patients on it for at least twelve months and found that prognosis of celiac disease was excellent: "There is complete recovery with no relapses, no deaths, no crisis, no pulmonary involvement and no stunting of growth."[8] By 1949, Dr. Sidney Haas's reputation was known throughout the world and on April 5th of that year, more than a hundred leading physicians met at the New York Academy of Medicine to pay him tribute. The New York Times reported:

> *Today, on the occasion of the fiftieth anniversary of his entrance into the medical profession, one of America's great pediatricians, Dr. Sidney V. Haas, is being honored for his pioneer work in the field of pediatrics. Among Dr. Haas's most important accomplishments was in the treatment of celiac disease, a digestive disturbance in which the child is intolerant of starchy food, and which was generally fatal at the time of his original work. Following his discovery that the carbohydrates in bananas could be tolerated by celiac patients, Dr. Haas developed an accepted routine therapy which laid the basis for later research and basic treatment in this field.[9, 10]*

In 1951, Dr. Haas, together with his son, Dr. Merrill P. Haas, published *The Management of Celiac Disease*, the most comprehensive medical text that had ever been written on celiac disease.[11] With 670 references to published reports, the book described celiac disease more completely than had ever been done before. The Drs. Haas presented their success with the Specific Carbohydrate Diet and offered their hypothesis in the last chapter of their book as to why the diet was effective. After decades of searching, it appeared that not only was an effective and lasting dietary treatment found, but that the Haas Specific Carbohydrate Diet was accepted by medical colleagues throughout the world as a cure for celiac disease.

But as Michael Crichton has written, "the battle" continued. Within one year after the publication of the Drs. Haas's book, a singular report appeared in the English medical journal, Lancet.[12] A group of six faculty members of the Departments of Pharmacology and of Pediatrics and Child Health of the University of Birmingham, after testing only ten children, decided that it was not the starch (carbohydrate) in the grains that so many had reported as being deleterious, but it was the protein, gluten, in wheat and rye flour that was causing celiac symptoms.

Gluten, like all proteins, is composed of hundreds of building blocks called amino acids which are linked together to form the protein molecule. In most people, the gluten molecule is broken down by digestive enzymes in the small intestine and the simple amino acids of which gluten is composed are absorbed by the intestinal absorptive cells to provide nutrition for the rest of the body.[13,14] It is believed that this is not the case in celiac disease and that the gluten remains undigested.

The Lancet report concluded:

> Gastro-intestinal function was investigated in ten children with coeliac disease. The changes were very similar to those in adult idiopathic steatorrhoea. The removal of wheat flour from the diet resulted in rapid improvement, both clinically and biochemically. Deterioration followed by reintroduction into the diet of wheat flour or wheat gluten, but wheat starch had no harmful effect.

They contradicted all previous work by stating that there was no need to restrict carbohydrates and, therefore, an unlimited choice of food could be ingested, provided that wheat and rye gluten were excluded. Further, "a high caloric diet may be given throughout with biscuits made from corn flour, soya flour, or wheat starch instead of wheat flour."

They maintained that it was not the starch in grains that was the culprit but it was the protein gluten and that when the gluten was "washed out" of the flour, the remaining starch was perfectly fine. And overnight, the hypothesis gained ready acceptance. No need now for doctors to worry about adhering to a diet which eliminated specific carbohydrates found in many foods; only one dietary exclusion would have to be made and that was the gluten in wheat and rye flour. It simplified the difficult problem of keeping people on a more restricted diet. No need to delve into food biochemistry and ask why gluten-containing foods such as corn would be permissible; it was to be a "black and white" remedy with no shades of grey.

Despite extensive research by many investigators, there is as yet no certainty about the precise nature of the gluten which is causing injury to the intestinal cells. During the 1970s, as newer techniques permitted researchers to further subdivide the large gluten molecule into smaller fractions, it was found that the alpha-gliadin fraction possessed toxic properties which appeared to injure intestinal cells of the true celiacs.[15] But there still remain unanswered questions about this smaller alpha-gliadin protein fraction: (1) is there a genetic lack of the digestive enzymes which would normally split these gliadin molecules into their single amino acids thereby preventing their harmful effects? (2) Is there a weakness in the membranes of the intestinal cells which permits the intact, undigested gliadin molecules to penetrate the intestinal cells and, once inside, "poison" the cells? (3) Do the gliadin molecules bind to the surface of the intestinal cells and, thereby, immobilize the cells and destroy them?

The most popular theory is that the gliadin fraction, by penetrating the intestinal cell membrane, reaches the underlying layer of white blood cells and causes an immune response. The products of the immune response, including antibodies, injure the intestinal cells and cause them to change their shape and to function abnormally.[15] More recent findings have implicated a carbohydrate molecule attached to the gliadin molecule as the toxic compound. When the carbohydrate is removed, the gliadin molecule is no longer injurious to the intestinal cells.[16,17]

Very recent research has cast more light on the gluten-celiac hypothesis and highlights the interaction between the starch and protein components of flour milled from grains. Almost all normal people fail to absorb a large amount of the starch of wheat flour.[18] This incomplete absorption of starch results in an increase in intestinal fermentation and the production of intestinal gas. In an effort to discover why wheat starch is not completely digested by many people, investigations were conducted relating to the physical structure of wheat flour. It was found that wheat flour is composed of granules containing a starch core surrounded by a network of gluten protein. This protein-starch complex can be separated by a manufacturing process whereby most of the gluten is removed. The remaining flour is sold as low-gluten flour and when it is substituted for regular wheat flour, there is improvement in starch digestion and absorption. Surprisingly, when the low gluten flour is baked into bread *together with the separated gluten,* starch malabsorption does not occur in spite of the fact that the same amount of gluten is present in the baked product as was present in the whole grain before gluten extraction. Since absorption of the wheat starch is complete, there is no resulting fermentation and intestinal gas. This indicates that it is not the gluten alone which results in intestinal symptoms.[18]

The investigators feel that it is the interaction between the starch and the gluten which results in the incomplete digestion and incomplete absorption of starch and which causes intestinal gas, abdominal discomfort, and diarrhea. They speculate that the gluten extraction process alters or exposes the starch core thereby making the starch more vulnerable to pancreatic digestive enzymes.[18,19] This intriguing interaction between the starch and protein of grains will, undoubtedly, be the basis for much future research and may be shown to have some bearing on those with celiac disease.

Some patients showed remarkable clinical improvement in their general well-being after following a "gluten-free" diet. However, biopsy samples, as viewed under the microscope, showed intestinal cells that were still markedly abnormal.[20] Additionally, some patients who started eating gluten suffered no ill effects at one time but became extremely ill at other times. Thus, not only do different celiac patients vary in their response to a gluten-free diet but the same patient may vary from time to time.[21] When the all-too-common relapse occurs, the patient is most often told that he/she must have inadvertently ingested gluten. It is common for patients to become so nervous about making a mistake that they assume that anything on a product that begins with "glut" must be gluten: glutamic acid, glutamine, monosodium glutamate, etc., or that gluten had somehow crept into the food in spite of the fact that it did not appear on the label.

It soon became apparent that grains which contained proteins other than gluten were having deleterious effects on the digestive tract. Some patients suffered relapses and exhibited damaged intestinal cells (microscopically) upon eating soy products.[22,23] Oats and barley were found to contain gluten-like proteins which offended many celiac sufferers.[24] Additional reports implicated rice as being harmful to intestinal cells.[25,26]

But the diet to manage celiac had been simplified and there now remained the problem of simplifying the diagnosis. The new diagnostic tool, the intestinal biopsy instrument, would be used to identify celiac. In spite of the symptoms the patient manifested, the patient would not be diagnosed as a true celiac until other criteria were met. A series of intestinal biopsies would be done: one tissue sample would be taken from the small intestine before gluten was removed from the diet; a second sample would be taken after the patient had been on a "gluten-free" diet. The biopsy samples would have to reflect the changes in the diet. When viewed under the microscope, the intestinal surface would have to appear flattened or blunted while the patient ingested gluten; after gluten withdrawal, the intestinal surface would have to revert to its normal architecture of "hills and valleys." If a patient fulfilled this established criteria, his condition would then be given the name, "gluten-induced enteropathy celiac disease." Thus, only a small number of persons exhibiting the clinical symptoms of malabsorption including diarrhea, bloated belly, and failure-to-thrive could now be classified as celiacs. The others, an even larger group, suffering with the same symptoms (but who did not pass the required test using the intestinal biopsy criteria) would be suffering from diarrhea from an unknown cause, steatorrhea (fat in the stool), malabsorption, sprue, etc. Therefore, if a physician applied the strict definition for diagnosing celiac disease, the number of "true" celiacs would remain very small while there would remain a large group of patients with assorted diagnoses or no diagnosis of any kind.[15] In a recent review of celiac disease, the gastroenterologist writing the article referred to this method of diagnosis as "the current gold standard for diagnosis."[27]

However, this method of diagnosis has been seriously questioned by a number of specialists. The flattened or blunted intestinal surface has been reported in innumerable disease states: infectious hepatitis, ulcerative colitis, parasitic infections of the intestine including various types of worms and one-celled parasites, kwashiorkor,[28] soy protein intolerance, intolerance to cow's milk protein, intractable diarrhea of infancy, Crohn's disease,[29] and bacterial overgrowth of the small intestine.[30] Bacterial overgrowth of the small intestine has also resulted in patchy broadening and flattening of the small intestinal surface. Just about all conditions associated with diarrhea seem to result in the same appearance of the small intestine as is seen in the so-called "true celiac."[24,25]

And in spite of increasing numbers of sophisticated tests developed to confirm the diagnosis of celiac including antibody tests, genetic testing involving HLA (histocompatibility antigens) markers, and twin studies, there appear to be more exceptions to the rule than those who "follow the rule." The reality is that thousands of patients are suffering and have never been given a diagnosis other than to see a psychiatrist, and thousands of patients are following "gluten-free" diets and are getting minimal relief, if any.

The most disquieting development in the gluten-celiac picture is the fact that celiacs, whether or not they respond favorably or unfavorably to gluten withdrawal, exhibit other serious intestinal problems which a gluten-free diet does not appear to be effective in preventing.[20,33] It seems, therefore, that something other than the protein, gluten, is involved in the underlying cause of the disorder.

Some investigators have always maintained that an inability to digest disaccharides induces the sensitivity to gluten.[34] But even were the disaccharides not the underlying cause of gluten intolerance, these double sugars should not be included in the diet of celiacs.[34] The flattened intestinal absorptive cells have lost their ability to perform the last step in digestion which is to split disaccharides.[29,35] Many researchers have confirmed the fact that in celiac patients, ability to digest disaccharides, especially lactose, is severely limited.[29, 36-38] To include disaccharides and certain starches in the diet of those exhibiting a flattened intestinal surface is to demand the impossible of these digestive and absorptive cells and to add to the existing problems.[39]

The following is part of an unsolicited letter sent to this writer and is, unfortunately, reported all too frequently.

> *After eight years of mysterious symptoms, dozens of doctors, gruelling, and often humiliating tests and general misery, no one could decide what was wrong with me. I discovered that because my two sisters and my daughter had been diagnosed as celiacs that I, too, should go on the gluten-free diet. Unfortunately, for both my daughter, another sister and I, the gluten-free diet did not work. Some symptoms were arrested but none of us were thriving and we just weren't absorbing food. We eventually found the Specific Carbohydrate Diet and it has been a godsend. I have never been healthier. My daughter, once a sickly (often whiney)*

withdrawn child with thin hair and dark circles under her eyes is outgoing, rosy-cheeked and happy. Everyone has noticed her thick, shiny hair. In fact she ran a marathon this year and placed 15th out of 79 children. Last year she ran the same race (before the diet) and placed 53rd, arrived weepy and slept all the way home in the car.[40]

I have been on the Specific Carbohydrate Diet for less than a year and still have a way to go but my life has changed drastically in this short time. Now I am actively pursuing my art interest—something I always had inside me, but didn't have the energy or drive to tackle.

The Specific Carbohydrate Diet has been shown to completely cure most cases of celiac disease if followed for at least one year. It is truly a gluten-free diet, eliminating all grains which contain gluten or gluten-like proteins while also recognizing the limitations of the injured intestinal surface. For those people who are not satisfied with their progress on the "gluten-free" diet, the Specific Carbohydrate Diet offers them the opportunity to become healthy.

Chapter 7

THE BRAIN CONNECTION

The search for the cause of schizophrenia and other serious neurological disorders, going back as far as the early 1900s, has led many investigators into the murky depths of the gastrointestinal tract. Although far removed anatomically from the brain, the intestine continues, now as it did then, to demand attention from the many researchers searching for the origin of neurological disorders. Repeatedly, the medical literature reports that allergists, gastrointestinal specialists, and psychiatrists have found that certain types of food, impaired digestion, and faulty absorption or ingestion of vitamins and minerals affect the function of the nervous system including the brain.

Celiac specialists, as early as 1908, had begun reporting evidence that some patients who suffered extended periods of diarrhea and malabsorption were also showing degeneration of the brain, spinal cord, and other groups of nervous tissue.[1] This deterioration of the nervous system in celiac disease was attributed to the patients' inability to absorb essential nutrients, including vitamins and minerals, due to injuries to the intestinal tract accompanying the disease.[1-3] As further advances were made in biochemistry and cellular biology, numerous scientific papers appeared showing, in great detail, the devastating effects of lack of certain vitamins and minerals on the brain and other nerve centers throughout the body.[4-5] Some forms of paralysis[1] and types of psychiatric disorders[4] were shown to be the result of nutrient deprivation which is known to be caused by malabsorption during intestinal disease. It has also been known for almost one hundred years that microbial action in the unseen world of the intestinal tract can be a source of toxins which affect normal brain function.[6-7]

When our younger daughter was cured of ulcerative colitis by dietary changes in the 1960s, the first symptoms to disappear were a type of seizures which occurred after she had fallen asleep. They were characterized by delirium, lasted about one hour and reoccurred several times weekly. Her recovery from the intestinal disease was preceded by an end to the seizures, never to return. During the seven years of doing consultations with people diagnosed as having Crohn's disease, colitis, and other forms of chronic diarrhea, I observed that improvement for many started with a disappearance of long-standing mental disorders including epilepsy, schizophrenia, mental confusion, poor memory, and bizarre behavior. And finally, with the distribution of my book, *Food and the Gut Reaction*, letters began arriving reporting this same phenomenon: mental disorders of long standing were clearing up even before the intestinal symptoms disappeared.

The medical literature abounds with published research which has attempted to explain this brain-bowel connection. The French scientist, Dr. H. Baruk, summarized fifty years of research on schizophrenia and mental disorders by stating:

> Instead of considering these illnesses hopeless, it is preferable to consider the majority of psychoses or neuroses as reactions to biological factors which are very often digestive in origin, and psychiatry must acknowledge them. These toxic factors are disregarded far too often.[6]

Baruk, as early as 1923, implicated a harmful strain of intestinal bacteria (E.coli, a normal inhabitant of the intestinal tract) as producing a toxin which exerts itself on the nervous system. This toxicity, Baruk concluded, produces a pathological sleep with delirium, resulting in psychotic-type mental confusion or schizophrenia.

About this same time period, the Drs. Buscaino of the Neurological Clinic of the University of Naples, Italy, reported that most schizophrenics showed some form of intestinal disease whereas manic depressive patients did not. Further, they found that the intestinal bacterial population of schizo-phrenics was abnormal. The Drs. Buscainos stated that:

> True schizophrenia (and not only some schizophrenic syndromes) appears to be the result of chronic intoxication from psychotoxic factors produced in the intestine.[7]

More recently, in the 1970s, a psychiatrist, Dr. F.C. Dohan, implicated all cereal grains and milk as being the dietary factors in this intestinal-brain connection.[8] Some investigators explained the adverse impact of these foods on mentally disturbed people as some sort of brain allergy or immune reaction, but there has been much controversy among scientists in their efforts to equate the effects of these foods with a typical allergic reaction. In 1991, Dr. J.O. Hunter presented his opinion on this controversial subject by writing that if this type of "food allergy" is not an immunological disease, but a disorder of bacterial fermentation in the colon, then it might be more appropriately named an "enterometabolic (intestinal) disorder."[9]

Dr. C. Orian Truss, an internist, has focused on the relationship of allergy and infection. With the publication of his book, *The Missing Diagnosis*, he launched the concept of Candidiasis (yeast infection) as being at the root of many types of mental as well as physical disorders.[10] Among many of his patients with innumerable symptoms, psychotic symptoms, including schizophrenia and neurosis, were often part of the picture. Based on the premise that the intestinal flora, yeast in particular, was in a state of imbalance (dysbiosis), he included in his treatment and cure a diet free of carbohydrates. Why? Because of all dietary components, undigested and unabsorbed carbohydrates (starch and sugar) have the greatest influence on the growth of intestinal microbes.[11]

In the late 1970s and through the 1980s, a number of reports were published in medical journals which added fuel to the burning issue of the bowel-brain connection. Doctors reported that among patients who had undergone surgical shortening of the small intestine (a treatment for serious gastrointestinal disorders as well as obesity), thereby decreasing their ability to break down and absorb food, patients were presenting with unusual neurological symptoms.[12-15] Among the symptoms were aggressiveness, sudden disorientation, blurred vision, blunted judgment, abusive behavior, slurred speech, staggering gait, rolling of the eyeballs, confusion, and delirium. The attacks lasted between 36-80 hours. Using the most sophisticated methods of analysis, it was found that carbohydrates were not being digested or absorbed (surgery had severely limited digestive capacity) and intestinal bacteria were, therefore, flooded with a surplus of carbohydrates which were being fermented in the remaining intact, intestinal tract. As a result, a waste product of bacterial fermentation, D-lactic acid, was being produced in abnormally large amounts.[16] It is currently thought that this acid, along with other toxic products produced by intestinal microbes, is entering the brain and "poisoning" the brain cells. Although the many patients exhibiting these symptoms have been treated with antibiotics to kill the bacteria producing the toxins, it has been stated that D-lactic acid is more effectively managed by preventing its formation, accomplished by manipulating dietary carbohydrates.[17] It has also been noted that this same type of malabsorption and the resulting production of D-lactic acid occurs not only when there has been surgical shortening of the intestine but in other gastrointestinal disorders as well.[18] In addition, it is a well known fact in veterinarian medicine that in cattle, D-lactic acidosis results from overfeeding with grain.[12]

Since the publication of my first book in 1987, numerous reports from individuals with both intestinal and neurological problems have been brought to my attention. The following are only a few case histories which show the dramatic relationship between intestinal and brain function:

A young woman with ulcerative colitis was reporting her symptoms to me when her Mother interrupted to tell me more. Apparently, the daughter was under the care of a neurologist (as well as a gastroenterologist) because she barked like a dog in her sleep. She had been taking a schizophrenic drug for this peculiar symptom. I was curious to check on this woman's progress with the Specific Carbohydrate Diet because of similar cases that had improved. When I called the day after her next appointment with the neurologist, she told me that her EEG (brain wave test) was normal for the first time in years. Shortly thereafter she was taken off the schizophrenic drug. It took longer for her ulcerative colitis to get better – about two years.

There have been many babies with chronic diarrhea accompanied by epileptic seizures. One baby was on commercial formula and was eating some solid foods. When his diet was changed to the Specific Carbohydrate Diet, both diarrhea and the epileptic seizures cleared up. He continues to do well six years later. Another baby with seizures was being breastfed and was also eating cereal. The Mother went on the Specific Carbohydrate Diet, the baby was allowed only those foods on the diet, and the epilepsy disappeared. He has been free of seizures for five years.

The following letter to a local newspaper further illustrates this bowel-brain connection. The letter was written in response to an earlier newspaper article relating to a young woman with Crohn's disease accompanied by mental symptoms. Upon calling the writer of this letter, other details were given: the writer's husband had spent forty years in and out of psychiatric institutions with the diagnosis of schizophrenia which accompanied his intestinal disorder.

The Cobourg Daily Star, **November 23, 1989**

Letters to the Editor

Diet held cure for deadly illness

Today I read with great interest and much sadness your article on Marilyn Isaac and the "mystery" disease with which she battled so long and so sadly lost.

My husband has suffered all his life from this disease, but unlike most he found help for his illness. Like Marilyn he was treated for mental disease and different illnesses for more than 40 years. His weight by this May had gone below 150 pounds. He had bled internally until he was too weak to move around and was vomiting continually, unable to keep food down. As his physical condition declined, his mental attitude declined as well.

I am an avid reader of your paper. Sometime in early May you had a column in your paper about a book written by Elaine Gottschall B.A., M.Sc. called **Food and the Gut Reaction.** She was in town at one of our health food stores. I bought the book, which was available at one of the book stores. It has been a miracle-the diet is not a hard one to follow, only requiring some extra food preparation, but well worth the effort.

By now, after four months of the diet, my husband has gained 40 pounds and is mentally well enough to drive his car, something he hasn't been able to do in years. He has been able to do all his own work and requires no help to care for me (I have been in bed for quite some years). I think, if you would use your article on this diet again, it might bring the worth of this diet to some other suffering individual. I thank you for taking the time to read this letter and maybe help others.

Betty Elder

Chapter 8

The Autism Connection

"....in many autistic children, bacterial and fungal overgrowths are etiologically significant in the cascade of events that result in autism or one of the other autism spectrum disorders."
by Jaquelyn McCandless in Children with Starving Brains.

"A sensible and harmless form of warfare on the aberrant population of intestinal microbes is to manipulate their energy (food) supply through diet... By depriving intestinal microbes of their energy source, their numbers gradually decrease along with the products they produce."
by Elaine Gottschall in Breaking the Vicious Cycle.

"Janie played with a doll for the first time ever today; I almost fainted. She initiated a hug and kiss for the first time ever in her 14 years of life."
From Mom of Janie with Down's syndrome, autism and gastrointestinal issues after a short time on the Specific Carbohydrate Diet.

The Specific Carbohydrate Diet has entered the world of autism through "the back door"– the intestinal tract. And what may have first appeared to be "the back door," via the digestive system, is rapidly becoming one of the most scientifically researched areas in determining what may be one of the underlying causes of many autism spectrum disorders.[1] Because the Specific Carbohydrate Diet's goal is to heal the intestinal tract and to rid it of bacterial and fungal over-growth, it is proving to be a very successful dietary intervention in treating many autistic children and leading them back to a life of normalcy.

This chapter will review some of the research dealing with the Gut-Brain Axis in child developmental disorders. It will point out how dietary intervention with the Specific Carbohydrate Diet addresses and often overcomes conditions thought to be at the root of autism spectrum disorders as well as some cases of epilepsy and attention deficit disorder (ADD).

Chapter 7, The Brain Connection, highlights the research of many years in which it had been shown that various neurological problems originate in the digestive system. And when the number of autistic children soared within the last two decades, attention has again been directed to the gastrointestinal tract.

Parents of autistic children have always known that, among their children's symptoms, there exists symptoms of chronic constipation, periods of diarrhea, and abdominal pain. But until recently, the parents' reports were treated as of no consequence. Now, fortunately, attention is being focused on these physical symptoms as well as on behavior, and many gastroenterologists are in agreement that "these children are ill and are in distress and pain, and not just neurologically dysfunctional."[2]

Some physicians, recognizing that diet was playing a part in causing the intestinal symptoms, focused their attention on treating these gastrointestinal symptoms as allergies and/or sensitivities. When testing these patients, they found evidence of sensitivities to various food components, mainly the gluten of grains and various components of dairy products. The behavior of many autistic children, although not all, showed improvement with the removal of these foods from their diet but, unfortunately, although behavior often improved, intestinal function did not. It was not unusual for the author to receive letters from parents as follows:

"My son is almost six years old and has autism. He was gluten/casein free for two years and while, during the first six months I thought I saw improvement in his exhibiting less stimmy (repeating the same action over and over again), his stimming returned. Even while on this diet, he still had constant stomach problems – being hospitalized four times for throwing up and dehydration. One time he suffered with a bowel obstruction; the other times they weren't sure what brought on his violent vomiting attacks. No doctor even bothered to do a colonoscope. I have mentioned to our doctor for years that he seems to be addicted to potato chips, french fries, ketchup, and waffles. When I learned of the Specific Carbohydrate Diet, it addressed this carbohydrate addiction and I intend starting this diet promptly."

And another letter from Patricia:

"...Meanwhile, my younger child's health was failing. He was on a strict gluten-free diet because of celiac disease. But it wasn't helping. He was ghost white and rail thin, with little energy and with chronic diarrhea and black circles under his eyes. Deep down, I worried he was dying. The team of pediatric specialists we were seeing had no clue how to make my little boy healthy, nor did my daughter's "alternative" DAN (Defeat Autism Now) physician. Fortunately, for us, this was August and every doctor treating my son was on vacation.

In desperation, I picked up a book called Breaking the Vicious Cycle: Intestinal Health through Diet *by Elaine Gottschall. A stranger had mailed this book to me two months earlier after meeting my Mother and hearing about my son's deteriorating health.*

The book explained why my son wasn't thriving on the regular celiac diet. His intestines were so damaged he couldn't digest any grains, or complex carbohydrates. The next day, he started the so-called Specific Carbohydrate Diet (SCD) described in this book. His stools became normal, and he

started growing and gaining weight. He's now a strong,
healthy seven-year old.

What about my daughter? She had no obvious digestion
troubles, but she did have "autism" and a recently discov-
ered yeast overgrowth. One British researcher found a link
between the MMR shot, intestinal problems, and autism.
Wouldn't a diet that promised to heal her intestines and
help with yeast overgrowth be her best shot at normal life?

We put Maria on a dairy-free version of the SCD. She had
a terrible yeast die-off that lasted a week even though she
was taking Nystatin, a popular antifungal drug. But once
she recovered from the die-off, about a week later, we were
confident she'd someday grow into an independent adult,
thanks to this remarkable diet. Her remaining speech pecu-
liarities, such as mixing up the order of words in a sentence,
disappeared. Her eye contact became normal. By the time
she was 4-1/2, one year after her diagnosis, no one would
guess she was ever "autistic."

These parents' reports are echoed throughout the autistic
community: although various dietary proteins appear to
aggravate behavioral symptoms, their removal is not address-
ing the gastrointestinal problems. In addition it becomes
increasingly apparent that as a few dietary proteins are
removed, more and more must be taken out of the diet to
hopefully achieve and sustain progress until these children
have little to eat in the way of nutritious food. Parents contin-
uously complain of their children's addiction to carbohydrates.

Dr. J. O. Hunter in 1991 described this dilemma of treating patients with gastrointestinal symptoms as food allergies or sensitivities. He stated that patients who exhibit
sensitivities do not follow classical Type I allergic reaction.
If these intolerances are not allergies, then they may be a
disorder of bacterial fermentation in the colon and the disorders
might be more appropriately named "enterometabolic (intestinal)
disorders."[3]

The Specific Carbohydrate Diet approaches these gastrointestinal challenges in autism as it has been successfully doing for inflammatory bowel disease – as a disorder of bacterial fermentation and the ensuing problems which occur because of bacterial fermentation. These problems resulting from bacterial fermentation are: (1) production of excess amounts of short chain volatile fatty acids (organic acids); (2) lowering of the pH of the blood as these acids are absorbed; (3) overgrowth of bacteria as the undigested carbohydrates provide food for bacterial proliferation; (4) mutation of some bacteria such as E.coli because of the change in pH in their colonic environment; and (5) excess toxin production caused by the overgrowth of some pathological bacteria.

Bacterial fermentation occurs when undigested carbohydrates escape digestion and absorption and end up in the lower parts of the small intestine and colon. Unlike diets that eliminate only certain proteins, based on tests showing sensitivities to proteins, and that allow unlimited intake of starches and sugars, the Specific Carbohydrate Diet (SCD) is designed to nourish the child optimally and to minimize bacterial fermentation.

Coleman and Blass in 1985 in *The Journal of Developmental Disorders* reported the first evidence that autism might be linked to carbohydrate metabolism (digestion).[4] These researchers reported that the syndrome of D-lactic acidosis was found to be present in autistic children. Their work was based on reports of the 1970s and 1980s showing that undigested carbohydrates were being changed by bacterial action in the intestine to a substance, D-lactic acid. High amounts of D-lactic acid in the bloodstream have been found to cause bizarre behavioral symptoms. This book discusses earlier research relating to D-lactic acidosis in Chapter 7, The Brain Connection.[5, 6, 7, 8, 9, 10, 11]

There are two approaches to treating this abnormal production of D-lactic acid: (1) use of antibiotics to kill the bacteria producing the substance, a method often used medically, and (2) decreasing the amount of fermentable carbohydrates upon which bacteria feed in order to produce

D-lactic acid. Since antibiotic therapy often is accompanied by other side effects, it seems reasonable to suggest dietary changes to accomplish the same thing or as a support for medical intervention with antibiotics.

The year 2000 yielded landmark research in linking autism to the gastrointestinal tract. It was reported that among 385 children on the autism spectrum, significant gastrointestinal symptoms occurred in 46% compared with only 10% of almost 100 children without autism, confirming what parents already knew.[12]

A flurry of remarkable scientific papers appeared, first, in the British medical journal, *Lancet*[13] and then in *The American Journal of Gastroenterology* (Wakefield)[14], demonstrating conclusively that serious intestinal pathology was found in more than half of autistic patients. These intestinal problems ranged from moderate to severe including esophagitis, gastritis and enterocolitis along with the presence of lymphoid nodular hyperplasia. Some of these intestinal pathologies resembled Crohn's disease as well as ulcerative colitis. As would be expected, from previous research done on intestinal problems (see pages 22–24), it was also found by Horvath et al[15] that there was low carbohydrate digestive enzyme activity (see diagrams of injured microvilli in the chapter on Carbohydrate Digestion), although the pancreatic function was normal.

Horvath's report concluded by saying unrecognized gastrointestinal disorders, especially reflux esophagitis and disaccharide malabsorption, may contribute to the behavioral problems of the non-verbal autistic patients.

Additional reports from findings at Harvard Massachusetts General Hospital conclusively showed that carbohydrate digestion is being hampered at the locus of the intestinal absorptive cell.[16]

Initial autism research findings at Harvard Massachusetts General, testing 400 autistic children, found that (1) lactase deficiency was found in 55% of ASD children tested; (2) combined deficiency of disaccharidase enzymes was found in 15%; and (3) enzyme assays correlate well with hydrogen breath tests. (The hydrogen breath test measures the amount of hydrogen gas given off when intestinal microbes ferment unabsorbed carbohydrates.)

This current work, on the decrease in the action of disaccharidase enzymes, leading to malabsorption, forms the basis for therapy of the Specific Carbohydrate Diet. Its goal is to keep disaccharide ingestion to a minimum by avoiding lactose, sucrose, maltose and isomaltose (remnants of starch digestion) and to provide a nutritious, healing diet without these double sugars. It deprives the microbial world of the intestine from a surplus of fermentable carbohydrates.

It is well known that compounds arising in the intestinal tract can enter the bloodstream and cross the blood brain barrier.[17] Gastroenterologists have been aware of this in treating the neurological effects of liver disease, hepatic encephalopathy. Reports have been published on how these toxins from the intestinal tract affect neurotransmitter substances in the brain.[18] Other research by E.R. Bolte[19], in an effort to correlate autism behavioral symptoms to the intestinal tract, investigated how the toxin of one bacterium, Clostridium tetani, could find its way from the intestinal tract to the central nervous system via the vagus nerve.

But there is still disagreement among researchers as to what constitutes the toxins from the gastrointestinal tract and what their origins are. Again, are they derived from proteins or are they products of intestinal bacterial action? This question was addressed in an outstanding research paper published in *Neuropsychobiology* in 2002 and authored by Dr. Harumi Jyonouchi et al.[20] Dr. Jyonouchi's group was the first to explain how bacterial toxins from the intestine can result in sensitivities to certain dietary proteins and casts light on the conundrum of which comes first: allergies/sensitivities which might lead to intestinal inflammation, or bacterial and yeast overgrowth (infections) which can lead to sensitivities to certain dietary proteins. The question can be viewed as "can the body's innate immune system, by reacting to the toxins of certain bacterial cell walls, cause the sensitivities to proteins such as casein and gluten?" The authors suggest that the root cause of the food protein sensitivity may be an underlying sensitivity to endotoxin, which arises from the surfaces of gram-negative bacteria in the gut flora: the lipopolysaccharide component of the cell wall of certain bacteria present in the intestine.[21]

This response, to an endotoxin of intestinal bacterial cells, is considered an innate immune response, an ancient form of defense coded in the genes as an inherited trait. This innate immune response to the bacterial toxin could stimulate the production of antibodies and cytokines, initiators of an inflammatory response, part of an adaptive immune response.[22] Dr. Jyonouchi's research is an attempt to answer the question of why there is gastrointestinal pathology in children exhibiting autism spectrum disorders and invites the research community to explore dietary intervention in order to ameliorate the behavioral symptoms of autism.

It is the hope of the author that this book will be of help to the research community in understanding how the molecular components of commonly eaten foods affect this problem and how changing the child's diet can, indeed, break the vicious cycle.

* *

Pamela Ferro, a registered nurse in private practice in Massachusetts, specializes in the treatment of children diagnosed with Autism Spectrum Disorder (ASD). She is also the parent of a child with autism. In treating over 300 children with ASD, she reports that at least 90% of these children present severe gastrointestinal problems that were unrecognized and, therefore, untreated. Her clinical experience shows that many of the behavioral symptoms associated with autism can be traced to an injured intestine. The Specific Carbohydrate Diet addresses the vicious cycle of malabsorption, maldigestion, inflammation, and food allergies seen in children with autism. Once healthy digestion begins, many children with autism demonstrate remarkable improvements in bowel function, language, eye contact, self-stimulatory behavior, anxiety, and mood. Ms. Ferro has developed a modified version of the Specific Carbohydrate Diet that eliminates the use of dairy for three to six months. As the child's behavior becomes stabilized, parents can slowly reintroduce dairy and evaluate whether or not it can be tolerated.

Note: The Specific Carbohydrate Diet was designed to treat bowel disorders and not specifically for ASD. Dairy is allowed on the Specific Carbohydrate Diet in the form of butter, certain cheeses and homemade yogurt. It not only adds variety to the diet, but homemade yogurt provides one of the best vehicles to introduce healthy bacteria into the bowel.

* *

Important note to parents of autistic children:

When implementing the Specific Carbohydrate Diet, it is important to remember that during the first week to ten days, profound changes are occurring in the digestive tract: the hundreds of different families of microorganisms are changing their metabolic functions due to the lack of nutrients to which they have been accustomed and of which they are now being deprived. Some children may do well even during the first week. But others will go through a period of adjustment which some refer to as "detoxification." It will be helpful during this period to find support from the many other parents who have been through this change. Going to the websites listed below can give you this support.

It is especially important that you read the information on these websites relating to the introduction of dairy products. A decision can then be made if the Specific Carbohydrate Diet should be implemented with or without dairy.

http://www.pecanbread.com

http://www.breakingtheviciouscycle.info
The ONLY official SCD website

Other websites, although not officially SCD, can be of great support to parents who are just starting the SCD commitment. Remember, advice from support groups differs and is subjective.

Chapter 9

INTRODUCING THE DIET

One basic principle of the diet must be firmly established and
persistently repeated: no food should be ingested that contains carbohydrates other than those found in fruits, honey,
properly-prepared yogurt, and those vegetables and nuts listed. While this principle may be clearly understood, it is sometimes difficult in practice to recognize the existence of
carbohydrates in various foods. Small quantities of carbohydrates other than those designated often creep into the diet
unless the strictest attention is paid to every item of food.[1]
Reading labels, although a good policy, is inadequate for
those on the Specific Carbohydrate Diet since one ingredient
sometimes has numerous names and may not be easily recognized as a forbidden carbohydrate. Many cans, jars, bottles,
and packages do not list all ingredients because of different
labeling laws in different parts of the country. *It is recommended that nothing be eaten other than those foods listed in
Chapter 10, The Specific Carbohydrate Diet.*
    Because fruits and raw vegetables have qualities which
tend to make them laxative, they must be used with care
when diarrhea is still active. Although all fruits, all raw vegetables, and as much honey as desired may be used when the
diarrhea has cleared, it is best to eliminate them until that
time. When fruits are introduced, after a week or two, they
should be ripe, peeled, and cooked. Raw fruits should not be
introduced until diarrhea is under control. Raw vegetables
such as salad greens, carrots and celery sticks, cucumbers, and
onions also should not be introduced until diarrhea is under
control.

Ripe, mashed banana is one of the uncooked fruits which may be tried first. Start cautiously with about one-quarter banana the first day. Only fully ripe bananas with no trace of green at the tips, the skin well-speckled with brown, and the edible portion soft enough to mash easily should be used. Most of the carbohydrate in the unripe banana is in the form of starch which is converted, in the process of ripening, to monosaccharide sugars which are easily absorbable by those with malabsorption problems.

Most canned fruits, or fruit packed in jars, are forbidden because of the added sugar. If cooked fruits are desired, they may be prepared at home with saccharin or honey. Artificial sweeteners other than saccharin should be avoided. It is interesting to note that saccharin has been vindicated as far as bladder cancer is concerned.[2]

Low calorie diet foods often contain sorbitol or xylitol as sweeteners. Occasionally low calorie diet chewing gum or candy containing these sweeteners may be used. However, excessive use of these products can cause diarrhea and bloating.[5]

The Specific Carbohydrate Diet includes dairy products although fluid milk and some commercial products are eliminated. A list of the many cheeses which are allowed can be found in the Appendix along with those cheeses which are not permitted. Homemade yogurt, prepared according to instructions found in the recipe section, is permitted. It is very important that the yogurt instructions be followed precisely so that virtually none of its lactose remains. This is particularly true for the length of fermentation; *a minimum of 24 hours is required.* Another dairy product which should be included is *dry curd* cottage cheese.* Every effort should be made to obtain this high-protein, sugar-free cheese for which the dairy man in your local market should help you find a source. It is not acceptable if it has any form of added milk or cream. Dry curd cottage cheese is a very important part of the diet since it may be "creamed" with homemade yogurt and

---

* NOTE: See Appendix for sources of dry curd cottage cheese.

substituted for regular cottage cheese. It may be used as a base for pancakes and cheese cake, and it may be used for short periods as an infant formula (see Gourmet Section).

WARNING: Some dairies are calling a type of cottage cheese (with added milk products) "uncreamed" since there is very little fat (cream) in the milk which has been added. This type of cottage cheese is **not** permitted. It is quite moist, contains a considerable amount of lactose, and should immediately be recognized as not being a **dry** curd.

It is not advisable to use lactose-hydrolyzed milk (LHM) either prepared in the home or as a commercially available product at the beginning of the dietary regimen. Although lactose-hydrolyzed milk decreases fermentation in the intestine, its effect on the liver of those with chronic intestinal disorders has yet to be investigated. Additional research should be conducted to determine the speed with which the sugars of LHM milk reach the liver. Only then will it be known if the blood galactose (one of the sugars in LHM) stays within normal levels or rises too high.[3] Once the individual makes considerable progress and is on the road to recovery, small amounts of LHM may be used in tea, coffee and in cooking.

When brisk diarrhea is no longer present, egg may be added to the diet. When bowel movements are formed and occur no more than two or three times daily, cooked vegetables may be added to the diet cautiously, one at a time, with a sufficient period between each new introduction to determine its effect. In some instances diarrhea recurs when vegetables or fruits are given, in which case their use must be postponed. In general, squash, tomato, string beans, and carrots, all in cooked form, are well tolerated. Canned vegetables, or vegetables packed in jars, are not permitted because many have added sugar or starch which the labels often do not indicate. Potatoes and yams are not permitted.

Fats in association with meats, in butter, cheese, and in homemade yogurt are well tolerated. It is usually not necessary to use skim or 2% milk unless one is eliminating fats in order to lose weight or because of some other health problem.

The Specific Carbohydrate Diet is highly nutritious and, depending on the choice of foods, is well-balanced. Every effort should be made to "round-out" the diet by eating sensibly and not, for example, consuming large quantities of meat or more than four muffins each day *to the exclusion of other foods.*

The diet should be discussed with your physician. Medication should continue as the physician has instructed. As progress is made, the physician, undoubtedly, will reduce medication gradually. WARNING: There are very specific procedures by which certain medications are reduced and it can be dangerous to discontinue their use improperly. Always seek medical advice in reducing medication.

As is advisable for all people, a daily diet should consist of a variety of foods: vegetables, fruits, cheeses, nuts, and some animal products. However, if one desires a diet without animal products, it is possible to eliminate them. The many essential nutrients which one gives up when on a strict vegetarian diet must be considered. It is beyond the scope of this book to include lists of foods which are rich in iron and B12, two nutrients which are difficult to get in a strict vegetarian diet, and it is the responsibility of those who choose vegetarianism to see that other foods replace the nutrients given up when one eliminates animal products. Since soy products, including tofu, are not permitted on this diet, it will be very difficult, but possible, for a strict vegetarian to obtain sufficient nutrients and calories.

Most people with chronic intestinal disorders also suffer from malabsorption and, consequently, are malnourished. It is advisable that they add a vitamin supplement that specifically states that it is free of sugar, starch, and yeast (see Appendix). It may be necessary to write to the company manufacturing the vitamin to be sure of the ingredients. Any supplement such as bee pollen or herbs must be carefully checked since many companies have used whey (70% lactose), sugars, or starches as fillers and binding substances.

In the winter, in northern climates, vitamin D should be taken in combination with vitamin A as cod-liver or halibut-oil (400 I.U. Vitamin D and 5000 I.U. Vitamin A). For people who cannot tolerate the oils, even in capsule form, there are excellent substitutes in the form of water-soluble Vitamins A and D.

The malabsorption of Vitamin B12 is very often a part of chronic intestinal disorders and a special effort should be made, often by injections by the physician, to bring B12 levels up to **high normal.** There is some evidence that low levels, although they fall within the "normal" range, are not ideal for optimal health.

The B-Complex vitamins: B1, B2, Niacinamide, B6, Pantothenic Acid, Folic Acid, Biotin, and B12 may be taken as a supplement (all in one tablet). Too much Folic Acid should be avoided; the amount taken should range from about 0.1-0.8 mg. Folic Acid and B12 work in unison in the cells of the body and it is important not to take more than 0.4 mg Folic Acid unless one is positive that B12 levels are in the high normal range; only then may one take up to 0.8 mg.

Any woman with an intestinal disorder who is on the contraceptive pill must very seriously consider vitamin supplementation, especially of the B-Complex family of vitamins, some of which are depleted by birth control medication.

Since Vitamin C is readily destroyed as a result of cooking and exposure to air, it is advisable that at least 100 mg be taken daily. If larger amounts of Vitamin C are currently being taken, one may continue provided that there is no starch or sugar in the Vitamin C preparation and that one is certain that the higher doses are not contributing to diarrhea.

It is the belief of the author that very large doses of added vitamins are unnecessary; the diet is highly nutritious and vitamin supplements are used in moderation to help in the recovery. Added minerals may be in order but it is very difficult to obtain satisfactory mineral supplements.

While cells of the body require approximately twenty different minerals, most mineral supplements contain only about eight. Since minerals compete with each other for absorption by the intestinal cells, it is possible that by taking a few, rather than all twenty, one could upset the delicate balance which, ideally, would be obtained from a nutritious diet. However, since many people with intestinal disorders are malnourished, it would be wise to check with your physician concerning the levels of the important minerals such as calcium, iron, iodine, and potassium. If mineral levels are low, they may be taken for a short time until malabsorption is corrected. Minerals, unlike vitamins, are not destroyed by air or temperature but can be lost in cooking water. Once malabsorption is corrected, the superb nutrition of the Specific Carbohydrate Diet should supply adequate minerals.

NOTE: Maintaining proper calcium levels is extremely important, especially in babies and growing children. The infant formula in the Gourmet Section provides calcium but not as much as is found in fluid milk or yogurt. Therefore, if the infant formula is used for more than two weeks, blood calcium levels should be checked periodically by a physician who may suggest calcium supplementation.

It is impossible to specify the exact amount of vitamin supplementation necessary for each individual. These formulations are offered as reasonable amounts. Please check with your doctor.

For children:

Vitamin A	5000 IU$^+$	Vitamin B1	1.5-5 mg
Vitamin D	400 IU	Vitamin B2	1.5-5 mg
(not when getting summer sun)		Niacinamide	10-20 mg
Vitamin E	10-30 IU	Pantothenic Acid	2-5 mg
		Vitamin B6	2-5 mg
Vitamin C	50 mg^{++}	Biotin	30-100 ug^{+++}
		Folic Acid	0.1-0.3mg
		Vitamin B12	0.6-3.0 ug

For adults:

Vitamin A	5000 IU	Vitamin B1	10-15 mg
Vitamin D	400 IU	Vitamin B2	10-15 mg
(not when getting summer sun)		Niacinamide	25-50 mg
Vitamin E	100 IU	Pantothenic Acid	10-15 mg
		Vitamin B6	10-15 mg
Vitamin C	100-500 mg	Biotin	100-200 ug
		Folic Acid	0.1-0.5mg
		Vitamin B12	100-200 ug

[+] International Units
[++] milligrams
[+++] micrograms

The listed values are approximations. It is sometimes diffi-cult to get all members of the B-Complex family in one tablet. However, never purchase a B-Complex vitamin with only B1, B2, and Niacin. The minimal members of the B-Complex family which should be included are B1, B2, Niacin, Pantothenic Acid and B6. It is wise to purchase the fat soluble vitamins (A, D, E) separately from other vitamins. Unless they are in separate containers, there is a tendency to contin-ue taking Vitamin D in the summer which should not be done unless the individual is housebound or gets very little exposure to the sun.

In prescribing this diet it is almost more important to stress what is not eaten than what is eaten. *Any cereal grain is strictly and absolutely forbidden,* including corn, oats, wheat, rye, rice, millet, buckwheat, or triticale in any form, whether as bread, cake, toast, zweiback, crackers, cookies, cereals, flour, or pasta (spaghetti, macaroni, or pizza). New grain substitutes are being placed on the market frequently. Some such as amaranth, quinoa, and cottonseed contain carbohydrates of unknown analysis and are not recommended while on this diet. Cereal bran, in any form, is strictly forbidden because its indigestible fiber provides an overload of carbohydrates which are ferment-ed by intestinal bacteria. In addition, most forms of cereal bran contain large amounts of starch.[4] White table sugar or brown sugar is forbidden as a sweetener or in forms such as candy, pastries, or breads.

The strictness of this diet cannot be overemphasized nor should the difficulty of adhering to it be minimized. Faithful observance requires intelligence and vigilance on the part of those taking care of the individual or on the part of the person who cooks for himself or herself. It is surprising how many times a child will manage, despite the best supervision, to get hold of forbidden food. It is equally surprising how many parents will decide, despite all warnings, that "just a taste" of ice cream, cookie, or candy will do no harm. Such infringements will seriously delay recovery and it is unwise to undertake this regimen unless you are willing to follow it with *fanatical adherence.*

Many people have approached the dietary program by planning to give it a one month trial. If followed carefully for only one month, there should be changes for the better. These improvements provide the encouragement and support needed to commit oneself for the necessary longer period. It is recommended that a chart be kept for this first month. Hang it in a convenient location, preferably the kitchen. Across the top of the sheet, list those symptoms which describe the condition such as gas, diarrhea, or nightmares. Down the side of the sheet, number each line for the days of the month. At the end of each day, fill in the chart. For example, "four +'s" could be used to describe a lot of gas for that day. If there is a little less the following day, "three +'s" could be filled in. At the end of the month, progress can be evaluated. At this point, a personal commitment can be made to continue for a year or more, depending upon the speed of recovery.

If you see no improvement after a one month trial, the diet will probably not work for you. It is your decision at this point to return to your old pattern of eating or to continue eating according to the outlined diet. Your decision, of course, will depend upon your overall state of well being.

At the beginning of the program, when symptoms such as diarrhea and cramping are severe, the following basic diet should be followed for about five days. In other cases, one or two days on this basic diet is sufficient. The amounts of the specified foods to be eaten depend upon the appetite of the individual; there is no restriction as to quantities eaten.

Breakfast: Dry cottage cheese (moistened with home-made yogurt).
Eggs (boiled, poached, or scrambled).*
Apple cider or other permissible juice (½ juice, ½ water). See Appendix re: juices.
Homemade gelatin made with juice, unflavored gelatin, sweetener.

Lunch: Homemade chicken soup including broth, chicken, pureed carrots (see page 89).
Broiled beef patty or broiled fish.
Cheese cake (see page 128) without lemon rind and baked to custard consistency.
Homemade gelatin.

Dinner: Variations of above

If a food specified in the diet is known to cause an ana-phylactic reaction (severe allergic reaction) eliminate it per-manently from the diet. If, in the past, an allowable food did not agree with you, eliminate it for a short time (about one week) and try it again in small amounts. If, after a week of elim-inating it, a food continues to cause problems, do not include it in the diet.

If you find it impossible to obtain the dry curd cottage cheese, substitute the cream cheese recipe (drained home-made yogurt) listed in the Gourmet Section.

When diarrhea and cramping subside, cooked fruit, banana, and additional vegetables may be tried. If they seem to cause additional gas or diarrhea when they are added to the diet, delay their use until later. As the individual begins to feel better, the rest of the diet may be introduced. Do not use vegetables in the cabbage family until diarrhea has

* *Avoid if diarrhea is very severe.*

substantially subsided. Dried legumes may be added cautiously after being on the diet for about three months.

Most cases begin to improve within three weeks after the dietary regimen has been started and improvement usually continues. At about the second or third month, there is sometimes a relapse even when the diet has been carefully followed. This can occur if the person develops a respiratory infection or for no obvious reason. Do not allow this to discourage you! Once the individual gets over this, improvement is usually steady with minor setbacks occurring occasionally during the first year.

Many cases of celiac disease, spastic colon, and diverticulitis appear to be cured by the end of a year. Other disorders such as Crohn's disease and ulcerative colitis take much longer with the minimum time of two years on the diet. A rule of thumb is to stay on the diet for at least one year after the last symptom has disappeared.

At that time, introduce one forbidden food at a time. It is advisable to add only one food per week, starting with very small amounts and increasing the amount as the week progresses. The next week, another food may be added. If these foods appear to be well tolerated, one may decide to return to a regular diet. If symptoms recur upon the introduction of a forbidden food, it is best to remain on the Specific Carbohydrate Diet longer.

It is hoped that no one who recovers from his or her problem by following the Specific Carbohydrate Diet ever returns to a diet high in refined sugar and refined flours. These are lacking or low in nutrients, will not nourish the immunological system adequately, and can make the individual more susceptible to intestinal infections. We kept our child on the diet for seven years although the symptoms had disappeared at the end of two. We enjoyed this way of eating and preferred to be cautious. Since Dr. Haas had died two years after the diet was initiated, we had no way of knowing the right time to go off the diet and, realizing how highly nutritious the diet was, we decided not to risk going off it too soon.

Chapter 10

THE SPECIFIC CARBOHYDRATE DIET ™

ALLOWABLE PROTEINS (Meat, fish, dairy products, etc.)
All fresh or frozen beef, lamb, pork, poultry, fish (including shellfish), eggs, natural cheeses (listed in Appendix), homemade yogurt made according to recipe in Gourmet Section, **DRY CURD** cottage cheese. Canned fish (canned in oil or water).

NOT PERMITTED
Processed meats such as hot dogs, bologna, turkey loaf, spiced ham, breaded fish, canned fish with sauces, processed cheeses (listed in Appendix), smoked meats (unless you know definitely that sugar has not been added at some stage in the smoking process). Most available smoked meats contain considerable amounts of refined sugar. In many parts of the country, abattoirs are available that will smoke meats according to your specifications. However, for those people who cannot get their meat smoked without sugar, ordinary smoked bacon may be eaten once a week if it is fried very crisply.

Most processed meats are not permitted since they contain starch, whey powder, lactose, or sucrose. It may be possible to obtain hot dogs and other processed meats without these additives and, if so, they may be included in the diet. NO CANNED MEATS PERMITTED.

ALLOWABLE VEGETABLES - Fresh or frozen (with no added sugar or starch). NO CANNED VEGETABLES, OR VEGETABLES PACKED IN JARS, ARE PERMITTED.
Artichoke (French but not Jerusalem), asparagus, beets, dried white (navy) beans, lentils, and split peas (dried legumes prepared according to instructions in Gourmet

Section), broccoli, Brussels sprouts, cabbage, cauliflower, carrots, celery, cucumbers, eggplant, garlic, kale, lettuce of all kinds, lima beans (dried and fresh), mushrooms, onions, parsley, peas, peppers (green, yellow and red), pumpkin, spinach, squash (summer and winter), string beans, tomatoes, watercress, turnips (may be tried after considerable improvement).

Snacks can include raw vegetables provided that diarrhea is not active.

NOT PERMITTED
Grains such as wheat, barley, corn, rye, oats, rice, buckwheat, millet, triticale, bulgur, spelt. (No cereals, bread, or flour made from these).
Potatoes (white or sweet), yams, parsnips, okra, chick peas, bean sprouts, soybeans, mungbeans, fava beans, garbanzo beans.
Amaranth flour, quinoa flour, chestnut flour or any newly-introduced grain substitutes such as cottonseed.
Wheat germ. Seaweeds.
Caution: Many recipes from other countries, such as couscous, contain grain-like ingredients which must be avoided.

ALLOWABLE FRUITS – Fresh, raw or cooked, frozen (with no added sugar), and dried. Canned fruits, or fruits packed in jars, which state "packed in own juice"; none canned in any other kind of juice. In sweetening cooked or raw fruits, use honey or saccharin. No other artificial sweetener but saccharin is allowed.

Apples, avocadoes, apricots, bananas (ripe with black spots beginning to appear on skin), berries of all kinds (including blueberries), cherries, fresh coconut or unsweetened shredded coconut, dates (only loose California dates are permitted; dates which stick together in a mass have had syrup or sugar added and are not permitted), grapefruit, grapes, Kiwi fruit, kumquats, lemons, limes, mangoes, melons, nectarines, oranges, papayas, peaches, pears, pineapples (glazed pineapple is permitted only if the glaze is the result of the drying of the natural sugars in the pineapple), prunes, raisins (preferably dark), rhubarb, tangerines.

Some people are allergic to sulfites and should avoid dried fruit to which these have been added. If there is no sensitivity to sulfites, this type of dried fruit may be used occasionally.

Dried banana chips are usually coated with corn syrup or refined sugar and should be avoided unless they are known to be produced without such additives.

ALLOWABLE NUTS – Purchased with or without shells.

Almonds, pecans, Brazil nuts, filberts (hazelnuts), walnuts, unroasted cashews, boiled chestnuts, peanut butter (without additives of any kind). Roasted peanuts in the shell may be tried cautiously after being on the diet about six months when diarrhea is gone. Avoid shelled peanuts as most have added starch. Nuts sold in salted mixtures are not permissable since most have been roasted with a starch coating.

NOTE: Finely ground up nuts will be referred to as nut flour in the recipes. Use nuts ONLY as nut flour until diarrhea has cleared up. Then, nuts may be used as a snack and should be chewed well.

ALLOWABLE BEVERAGES (See Appendix)
JUICES

Canned tomato juice is permissible (only salt added). V-8 is not permitted because it contains added tomato paste, which is not allowed.

Use tomato juice for cooking *instead* of canned tomato paste, canned tomato sauce, or canned tomato puree. Avoid canned tomato juice mixtures such as tomato juice cocktail or other tomato juice mixtures.

Orange or grapefruit juice, freshly squeezed or juices, if available, not made from concentrate. All of these without added sugar. While diarrhea is active, AVOID ORANGE JUICE IN THE MORNING. If taken in the morning, it tends to increase diarrhea. However, it appears to be well tolerated later in the day.

Grape juice, white or dark. Bottled grape juice usually has no added sugar; avoid frozen grape juice which usually does have added sugar.

Pineapple juice (canned, frozen, or fresh) without added sugar.

Apple juice, formerly an allowable beverage, has become a problem because some manufacturers are adding corn syrup and sugar which is not listed on the label. Therefore, choose an apple *cider* packed by a local company you feel is responsible. You can call or write to them to ensure that it is pure apple cider without added sweetener. A preservative such as sodium benzoate is permissible. It is still possible in many areas to obtain freshly pressed apple cider and freeze enough for a year (Caution: fill containers only two-thirds full).

Juices packed in boxes, even those which state that there has been no sugar added, should be avoided since experience has shown that they are not well tolerated by those on the Specific Carbohydrate Diet.

Freshly squeezed vegetable juices of any of the allowed vegetables.

OTHER BEVERAGES

Weak tea or very weak coffee, perked or dripped, without milk or cream.

Some herb teas can be laxative. Restrict the use of herb teas to peppermint and spearmint.

Milkshakes made with homemade yogurt, fruits, sweetened to taste with honey or saccharin.

NOT PERMITTED

Fluid milk of any kind.

Dried milk solids.

Commercially prepared acidophilus milk which contains unfermented milk along with the acidophilus bacteria; much lactose remains.

Commercial buttermilk, commercial sour cream, or commercial yogurt (except for use as a starter for your own

homemade yogurt). Some companies are producing sour cream which contains virtually no lactose. Inquire concerning the availability of this permissible product in your area.
Enzyme-treated milk, except as noted in Chapter 9; milk drunk along with lactase enzyme replacement (in vivo replacement).
Soybean milk.
Instant tea or coffee.
Coffee substitutes; most have malt added which is not permitted.
Postum.

ALLOWABLE CONFECTIONS
A person on the Specific Carbohydrate Diet does not have to be denied sweets and other confections. With the use of honey, nuts, dried fruits, the most delicious cakes, cookies, muffins, and candies may be made.

ADDITIONAL INSTRUCTIONS
Although grains are not permitted, salad and cooking oils made from grains may be used; therefore, corn and soybean oils are permitted. Other oils which may be used for salads and cooking are sunflower and safflower oils. Olive oil is highly recommended.

Thicken gravy with boiled onion pureed in blender or with homemade mayonnaise (see Gourmet Section for gravy).

Unflavored gelatin is to be used for gelatin-type desserts.

Mustard is permissible; use plain mustard since gourmet types have many added ingredients which must be avoided.

Dill pickles and olives are permissible. Read labels carefully and avoid those with added sugar.

Vinegar is permitted (cider, white, or wine). Some gourmet-type vinegars have added sugar and should not be used.

Diet soft drinks are permitted occasionally. Those sweetened with aspartame or Nutri-Sweet may sometimes contain lactose and should be avoided, if possible. However, if this is the only type available, one per week is permitted. Diet soft drinks sweetened with saccharin need not be limited to only one a week: 2-3 weekly would be permissible.

DO NOT USE DIET SOFT DRINKS SWEETENED WITH ANY OTHER SWEETENER–some can aggravate intestinal problems to a great extent. Bottled water without any additive is permissible but those which have been marketed as "sport drinks," or have added fiber, vitamins, or minerals should be avoided. Soft drinks sweetened with FRUCTOSE and/or GLUCOSE should not be used (see next page).

Use butter, not margarine. Margarine contains added milk solids and/or whey. Cultured butter, if available, is highly recommended.

Spices of all kinds may be used. Avoid mixtures such as "apple pie spices" and curry powder; buy spices such as cinnamon and nutmeg separately.

Use fresh garlic and onions instead of garlic and onion powders which may have a starch base.

Coconut milk and almond milk may be tried after three months, if homemade. (See Gourmet Section).
CAUTION: If eating baked goods with almonds, consumption of almond milk should not exceed 8 oz (250 mL) daily.

Pasta such as spaghetti and macaroni is made from grains and is forbidden. There are substitutes for pizza and spaghetti in the Gourmet Section.

Do not use cornstarch, arrowroot starch, tapioca starch, sago starch, or other starches of any kind.

Do not use chocolate or carob.

Do not use bouillon cubes or instant soup bases.

DO NOT USE PRODUCTS MADE WITH REFINED SUGAR. This eliminates many commercially prepared products, some of which are listed in the Appendix.

Do not use agar-agar or carrageenan.

Do not use pectin in making jellies and jams (see recipes for jams in Gourmet Section).

Ketchup is almost 40% sugar and is not permissible. (see Gourmet Section for a quick ketchup).

No ice cream unless you make your own. Commercial ice cream is very high in lactose and sucrose. Even those commercial ice creams made with honey are often high in lactose.

No molasses, corn syrup, or maple syrup.

HONEY – This is the sweetener of choice. Although many health claims are made for various enzymes, pollen and other substances to be in the honey, it is preferred that, when on this diet, you use a honey which is fairly clear when held up to light. A slightly cloudy appearance is all right. Pasteurized honey from the store as well as honeys bought from a beekeeper are fine.

Do not use flours made from beans or lentils since beans and lentils were probably not soaked prior to grinding and in the dried form, they have too high a concentration of starch. Soaked and cooked navy beans (see instructions in Gourmet Section) may be drained and pureed and used in some of the cake recipes as an "extender" in order to cut back on the quantity of nut flour required.

Do not use baking powder. Use baking soda where specified.

Do not use seeds of any kind until three months after the last symptom has disappeared and then try them cautiously.

Although all natural cheeses may be used (see Appendix), there are two cheeses which are considered natural which must be avoided. They are Ricotta and Mozzarella. The brown, caramelized cheese called Gjetost must also be avoided.

Many medications have added carbohydrates of the wrong kind (sucrose, lactose and starch). Some of these medications may be obtained without these sugars by asking your pharmacist. The pharmacist may substitute and replace these with either fructose or dextrose. He may suggest the same drug but a brand made without lactose and sucrose. However, if the medication is only available with these added carbohydrates, use the medication when essential.

However, for your own consumption and food preparation, DO NOT USE FRUCTOSE OR GLUCOSE SYRUP NOR POWDERED OR GRANULATED FRUCTOSE, GLUCOSE OR DEXTROSE. Although they sound as though they are monosaccharide sugars, in recent years companies are selling them as a mixture of assorted sugars and still retaining the labeling of the single monosaccharide sugars. In other words, they are being mislabeled.

Do not use any product which contains FOS (fructooligosac-charides). This form of starch (inulin) may feed harmful bacteria as well as "friendly" bacteria and will defeat the benefits of the diet.

If you are using preparations containing "friendly" bacteria (which often contain other ingredients), it is better to use products that contain lactose (or whey) than FOS.

ALCOHOLIC BEVERAGES
Avoid beer.

Very dry wine is permissible. If a sweeter wine is desired, add a crushed saccharin tablet or sweeten with honey.

Occasionally gin, rye, Scotch, bourbon, vodka, etc. No sherry, cordials, liqueurs, or brandy.

Club soda is permissible as a mixer since it has no added sugar.

The following is a sample day's menu. The quantity of foods eaten should depend upon appetite. It is presented to give an idea of how the Specific Carbohydrate Diet can be implemented.

BREAKFAST
Baked apple sweetened with honey, if desired; cinnamon to flavor
Scrambled eggs
Homemade nut muffin with butter and homemade jam
Weak tea, coffee, grape juice, or apple cider

LUNCH
Tuna fish salad made with homemade mayonnaise, garnished with olives, dill pickle, on a bed of lettuce
Slices of cheddar cheese

Homemade pumpkin pie (recipe in Gourmet Section); nut crust can be used or the filling can be eaten as a pudding
Pina Colada made according to recipe in Gourmet Section

DINNER

Homemade spaghetti sauce made with ground beef, onions, garlic, herbs, tomato juice. Serve on a bed of boiled beans or spaghetti squash
Freshly grated cabbage salad with homemade mayonnaise or oil and vinegar
Peas and carrots with butter
Fresh fruit or cheese cake (recipe in Gourmet Section)
Tea

There is no specified schedule for introducing foods with the exception of homemade yogurt (See Gourmet Section). Some people may appreciate suggested guidelines but they are not generally required. The basic rules given in Chapters 9 and 10 are usually sufficient: For example, fruits (other than banana) should be peeled and cooked well. The order for introducing them and some of the vegetables varies with each individual. Going slowly and carefully is best determined by an individual's reactions. This the sensible approach endorsed by the author.

Websites which offer prepared SCD foods MUST be used with caution. Fruit bars, candy bars, juice extracts, etc. are rarely 100% SCD legal. Often, it is impossible to find out what the manufacturers of these products are doing. Also, methods and formulas can be changed without notice. It is best to prepare all foods in the home. Hiring a responsible person to come into your home once a week to bake and freeze entrees and baked goods is a good option to relieve the burden of work at the start. Many SCD foods such as ketchup and mayonnaise, baked goods and treats, can be made in a few hours and will last through the week. Larger quantities of many items can be frozen in small individual portions.

GOURMET SECTION

TABLE OF CONTENTS

APPETIZERS, DIPS, AND SPREADS

Apple-Raisin Peanut Butter Spread

This spread may be used on slices of cheddar cheese or as a dip.

¹/₂ cup peanut butter
(no additives)
¹/₂ cup unpeeled, diced apple

¹/₄ cup raisins
¹/₂ teaspoon ground cinnamon

In a small bowl sir together peanut butter, apple, raisins and cinnamon.
If too stiff to spread, add a little apple cider and blend ingredients together.

Liver Paté

1 lb. tender liver
(chicken or calf)
¹/₄-¹/₂ cup homemade
mayonnaise (see pg. 98)

1 small onion, cut into small
pieces
salt and pepper to taste

Pan fry liver in butter until it has lost its pink color.
Cool liver and cut into small pieces.
Place liver, onion, and mayonnaise in blender or food processor. (If using blender, place mayonnaise at bottom so that blades will turn easily.)
Blend until smooth.
Serve as a stuffing for celery, on lettuce leaves, or as a dip with raw vegetables.
Can be spread on squares of cheese and served as an appetizer.

Party Cheese Dip

1¹/₂ cups cheddar cheese, grated
¹/₄ cup soft butter
¹/₄ teaspoon dry mustard pow-
    der

¹/₃ cup apple cider or dry white
    wine
fruits such as apple or pear
    wedges or raw vegetables

Cream the butter; blend in mustard powder or cider.
Add the grated cheese and blend thoroughly.
Chill overnight, if possible, to blend flavors.
Allow to stand at room temperature for ½ - 1 hour.
Use with fruits or vegetables.

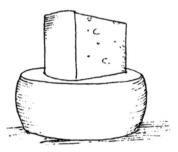

SOUPS

Carrot Soup

2 lbs. carrots, scrubbed and quar-
  tered lengthwise
4 cups homemade chicken stock
1 cup finely chopped onion

2 small cloves garlic, crushed
1 cup homemade yogurt
⅓ cup chopped almonds
3-4 tablespoons butter

Salt chicken stock to taste
Parboil carrots in chicken stock about 12-15 minutes. Cool.
Sauté the onion, garlic, chopped almonds in 3-4 tablespoons butter until tender but not browned.
Purée carrots, stock, sautéed mixture, and yogurt in a blender until smooth.
Add seasoning of your choice†.
Heat very slowly in a double boiler or chill and serve cold.
Garnish with toasted nuts, parsley or cress.

†Suggested seasoning combinations from which to choose:
1. Pinch nutmeg, ½ teaspoon mint, dash of cinnamon, OR
2. ½-1 teaspoon thyme, ½-1 teaspoon marjoram, ½ -1 teaspoon basil, OR
3. 1 teaspoon freshly grated ginger root sautéed in butter.

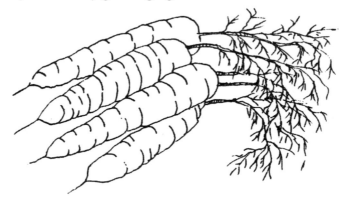

Cream of Tomato Soup

2 cups tomato juice   *honey or saccharin to taste*
1/2-1 cup homemade yogurt (see
*   pg. 157)*

Make a paste with the yogurt and ¼ cup tomato juice.
Slowly stir in the remaining juice.
Heat over low heat or in a double boiler, stirring occasionally.
Season to taste with salt, pepper, sweetener, and herbs of choice.

Gazpacho Soup

4 cups tomato juice   *juice of 1 lime (optional)*
1 small well-minced onion   *2 tablespoons white vinegar*
2 cups diced fresh tomatoes   *1 teaspoon tarragon (optional)*
1 cup minced green pepper   *1 teaspoon basil*
1 cup diced medium cucum-   *¼ cup freshly chopped parsley*
*   ber(peeled)*   *2 tablespoons olive oil*
1 clove garlic, crushed   *salt and pepper to taste*
juice of 1/2 lemon

Garnish: 1 hard boiled egg yolk chopped with a little parsley
(optional).

Combine all ingredients.
Chill for at least two hours before serving.
Note: Ingredients may be processed in a blender instead of
chopping separately.

Hearty Vegetable Soup

1 cup chopped celery
1 cup chopped carrots
1 cup chopped onion
¹/₂ cup chopped cabbage
2 cups tomato juice or a few
 fresh tomatoes
2 cups homemade chicken or
 beef stock OR

4 cups water and about 1 lb.
 beef bones
 (or ¹/₂-1 lb. beef)
2 tablespoons oil or butter
Season to taste (herbs and
 spices such as basil, salt,
 pepper, bay leaf)

If a food processor is available, all vegetables may be chopped in a few minutes using the steel blade.
Sauté onions and carrots in oil or butter until soft.
Add all other ingredients and simmer for 2 hours if stock is used; for 3-4 hours if beef bones or beef is used.

Chicken Soup

Using the largest pot you have, fill half of it with chicken parts (legs and thighs make the most flavorful soup).
Peel about ten carrots and add to chicken.
Add about two large onions, a few stalks of celery, and some parsley.
Season with salt.
Fill pot with water.
Simmer for about 4 hours and then strain soup through a colander or strainer.
Skim off top layer of fat (don't worry if you can't get it all).
Puree carrots in blender and return to broth.
Remove skin from chicken parts and return to broth.
Onions, celery, and parsley should not be used at the start of the dietary regimen because the fibrous parts of these vegetables may cause problems.

Roasted Eggplant Soup

This soup is a real gourmet treat.

2 medium eggplants
1 medium onion, sliced
2 stalks celery, roughly chopped
1 medium carrot, roughly
*   chopped*
1 tablespoon olive oil

4 cloves fresh garlic, minced
2 cups homemade yogurt
2 quarts chicken or shrimp
*   stock*
3 tablespoons butter
3/4 cup fresh basil
salt and pepper to taste

Slice eggplants lengthwise and rub with olive oil.
Place into a preheated oven (400°F, 200°C) until soft and golden brown.
In a large pot, combine onion, carrot, celery, garlic and stock and bring to a boil.
Reduce temperature and simmer until vegetables are tender.
Peel eggplant and cut into cubes.
Strain vegetables and return stock to pot.
Combine strained vegetables with cubed eggplant and purée in blender or food processor.
Add yogurt and butter to puréed vegetables and blend again in blender or processor.
Add vegetable and yogurt mixture to stock.
Heat gently to simmer stage.
Season with salt and pepper to taste and serve piping hot garnished with chopped basil.

(Recipe courtesy of David J. Couture)
(Submitted by Barbara Scheuer)

CONDIMENTS, SALADS,
AND SALAD DRESSINGS

CONDIMENTS

Chili Sauce

*1 – 6 qt. basket ripe tomatoes,
  unpeeled, chopped
6 cups celery, chopped
4 cups onions, chopped*

*2 cups green peppers, chopped
2$^{1}/_{2}$ cups vinegar
1 tablespoon salt
3 cups honey
dash of pepper*

All ingredients may be chopped very quickly in a food processor.
Combine all ingredients.
Bring to a boil in a large pot, stirring more often as the chili sauce
thickens. STIR FREQUENTLY to prevent scorching.
Simmer for about 30 minutes depending upon thickness desired.
Cool. Pack in plastic containers and freeze OR bottle and seal.

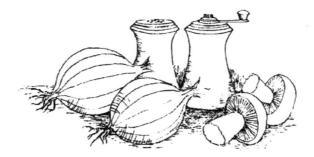

Honey-Ginger Chutney

1¼ cups honey
1 cup cider vinegar
6 or 7 cooking apples
2 lemons
2 green peppers or sweet red peppers
3 medium onions

1½ cups canned crushed unsweetened pineapple, including juice
1 cup raisins
4 teaspoons fresh ginger, grated
¾ cup almonds, slivered

Heat the honey and vinegar in a large saucepan,
Peel, core, and dice apples finely.
Add apples to the honey and vinegar and simmer for 20 minutes.
Remove the seeds and chop peppers and lemons finely, preferably in a food processor using the metal blade, and add to apple mixture.
Stir in the finely chopped onions.
Add the pineapple, raisins and ginger.
Simmer for 20 minutes more.
Add the slivered almonds and simmer for 30 minutes, stirring frequently to prevent sticking.

Ketchup

2 cups tomato juice
1-3 tablespoons white vinegar
honey and/or saccharin to taste
bay leaf (optional)
salt and pepper to taste

Mix all ingredients except sweetener and simmer on stove until thick, stirring often to prevent sticking.
When almost the desired thickness, add sweetener to taste and complete cooking.
Ladle into sterilized jars and seal immediately OR place in small containers and freeze.

Pineapple Cilantro Salsa

This recipe is a creation of Linda Hanson, CEO of Friseé, "Caterer of the Stars".

1 small, ripe pineapple	*¹/₂ red bell pepper*
1 small red onion	*salt and pepper to taste*
2 bunches of cilantro	

Peel and core pineapple.
Finely chop all ingredients starting with the pineapple.
Combine the finely chopped pineapple with one half of the red pepper and one half of the red onion.
Season with salt and pepper to taste and then add the fresh cilantro leaves that have been washed and finely chopped.
Depending on taste, add some of the remaining chopped onion and red pepper.
This salsa is especially delicious served with grilled chicken breasts, grilled white fish or salmon.
Fresh mango or papaya can also be chopped and added.
Some of the cilantro can be replaced with fresh mint leaves which have been finely chopped.

Raw Cranberry Relish

1 lb. fresh cranberries	*1 apple*
1 orange	*honey*

Wash and drain cranberries.
Cut orange into small pieces and remove seeds (orange need not be peeled).
Core apple and cut into small pieces.
Combine ingredients and process using blender, processor, or hand grinder until well mixed.
Sweeten to taste with honey.
Serve with meat or poultry or mix with dry curd uncreamed cottage cheese and serve on lettuce.

SALADS

Cottage Cheese Salad

1 cup uncreamed cottage cheese   ¹/₄ cup unsweetened pineapple
   (dry white curd)   (fresh or canned) or other
¹/₄ cup homemade yogurt   fruit in season

Mix ingredients together and serve on lettuce.

Halloween Carrot Salad (Pumpkin Heads)

2 cups grated raw carrots
¹/₂ cup homemade mayonnaise
lettuce leaves

Garnish: a few dark raisins and strips of green pepper

Mix carrots with mayonnaise.
Fill a small cup with carrot salad and unmold onto a lettuce-covered plate.
Make eyes and nose of pumpkin head using raisins.
Use strip of green pepper for mouth.

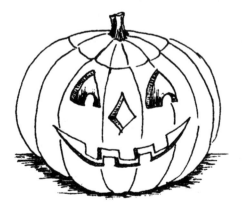

Mock Antipasto Salad

1 can anchovies
1 or 2 hard boiled eggs, quar-
    tered
2 fresh tomatoes, diced or sliced

lettuce, shredded
Italian herbs (oregano, basil),
    if desired
Oil and vinegar dressing

Mix all ingredients and chill.

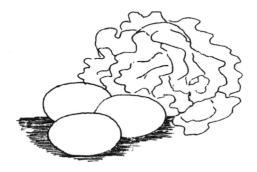

Seafood Salad

1 can tuna, salmon, or crab-
    meat or 1 lb. cooked and
    chilled bland fish (sole,
    halibut, cod, etc.)

1/2 cup homemade mayonnaise
lettuce leaves

Drain oil or water from canned fish.
Flake fish with a fork.
Add as much mayonnaise as desired, mix thoroughly, and chill.
Heap onto a bed of lettuce.

Summer Fruit Terrine

2 cups apple cider
2 envelopes unflavored gelatin
¼ cup honey
½ teaspoon vanilla (optional)
Fresh fruit:
   3 or 4 different kinds such as strawberries,
   raspberries, cantaloupe, honeydew melon, orange sections.

A standard-sized bread loaf pan is suitable for this recipe.
Apple cider, which is usually easier to buy in the Fall of the year depending upon where you live, can be frozen and then used during the summer months when fresh fruit is available.
In the top of a double boiler, heat the apple cider and honey.
Place gelatin in ½ cup cold water for a few minutes to soften.
When the cider is hot, add softened gelatin and mix thoroughly.
The amount of fruit used should be determined by the size of the pan.
Place a layer of fruit in the bottom of the pan and cover with cider. Refrigerate until firmly set.
Place another layer of fruit on top of first layer and cover with *cooled* cider. Refrigerate until second layer sets.
Repeat this process until loaf pan is full.
The gelatin layer between fruit layers should be at least ¼"- ½" thick.
Refrigerate overnight.
To remove, rub pan with a hot cloth on bottom and sides and invert on a serving dish.

(Recipe courtesy of David J. Couture)
(Submitted by Barbara Scheuer)

Waldorf Salad

3 cups apples, cut in chunks or
  ¹/₂ inch cubes (peeled or
  unpeeled)
1 cup pineapple chunks (fresh
  or canned, unsweetened)
¹/₄ cup raisins

1 stalk celery, chopped
¹/₂ cup thinly-sliced green pepper (optional)
1 cup thinly-sliced raw carrots
  (optional)
¹/₄ -¹/₂ cup walnut pieces

Combine all ingredients.
Blend with 1 cup of yogurt dressing or mayonnaise.
Serve on lettuce leaves.

Zucchini and Tomato Salad

2 cups diced uncooked zucchini
  or cucumber
2 cups diced fresh tomatoes
  (include juice)
¹/₄ cup chopped green onion

1 small green pepper cut into
  narrow ribbons
1 stalk celery, chopped
vinaigrette dressing

Prepare vegetables and add dressing.
Chill in refrigerator for one hour before serving.

SALAD DRESSINGS

Mayonnaise

May be made in a blender or food processor (using steel blade), If made in processor, recipe can be doubled. However, the recipe cannot be doubled if a blender is used; it will not thicken properly.

1 whole egg
1-1¼ cups oil
1 tablespoon white vinegar or fresh lemon juice
¼ teaspoon dry mustard powder

salt and pepper to taste
1 crushed saccharin (¼ grain)
or a little honey (optional)

Any vegetable oil or a combination of oils may be used.
Process in blender or processor for a few seconds: egg, lemon juice (or vinegar), and mustard.
While the machine is running, add the oil in a fine stream.
Do not add oil quickly; it should take at least 60 seconds.
As mayonnaise thickens, the sound of the machine will deepen.
With the machine running, add the mustard powder, sweetener, and other seasonings

Suggestions:

Use to thicken gravy: Add 2 tablespoons mayonnaise to about 1 cup of gravy liquid and heat gently for about 1 – 2 minutes, stirring constantly.

Use as a base for tartar sauce by adding ½ cup chopped dill pickles (unsweetened) and ¼ chopped onion.

Use as a mock Hollandaise sauce by adding grated cheddar cheese: Spread on vegetables such as cooked cauliflower or broccoli. Cover and heat on oven.

Mix with yogurt (1 part mayonnaise, 1 part homemade yogurt) and use as a salad dressing.

Vinaigrette Dressing

May be used for salads or for marinating chilled vegetables.
Combine in a small bowl:

¹/₄ teaspoon salt
¹/₄ teaspoon pepper
1 tablespoon olive oil

1 tablespoon vinegar or lemon juice
¹/₄ teaspoon dry mustard powder

Beat these ingredients well with a fork or a whisk until blended.
Add:

1 tablespoon vinegar or lemon juice

3 tablespoons olive oil
1 whole clove garlic, peeled

Store in a covered jar in a cold place until ready for use.
Shake well before using.

Yogurt Salad Dressing

May be used for fruit salads or vegetable salads

1 cup homemade yogurt
Juice of 1 lemon
Honey or crushed saccharin

Mix yogurt and lemon juice and sweeten to taste with liquid
honey or crushed saccharin tablets.

VEGETABLES

Baked Acorn (Pepper) Squash

1 acorn squash
a little butter
a little honey

grated orange rind
(¹/₄ teaspoon for each squash half)

Cut acorn squash in half and use ½ squash for each serving.
Scoop out seed cavity of each squash half.
Place cut side down on a cookie sheet and bake at 400°F (200°C) until a dull knife goes through squash easily.
Turn face up and dot with butter, honey, and grated orange rind. Return to oven and bake another 15-30 minutes at 350°F (180°C).

Variation: These squash "boats" may also be filled with a mixture of cooked poultry or cooked meat which has been mixed with vegetables and moistened with broth, yogurt, or onion gravy (see pg. 107).

Butternut Squash Slices

1 butternut squash
small amount butter
salt to taste

Slice the neck of a butternut squash (not necessary to peel). If crispness is desired, slice very thinly, about ¼" thick. If cut thin, these may be used as a substitute for French-fried potatoes.
Place on cookie sheet or pizza pan, dot with butter, and bake in a hot oven 450°F (230°C) until one side is brown.
Turn and brown other side.

Carrot Curls

This recipe may be used as a substitute for potato chips or when something crisp is desired.
Using a potato peeler, make curls out of about 3 carrots.
Deep fry in oil until they turn golden brown.
Drain in a colander or strainer. Refrigerate oil for next batch. (Do not use oil more than 3 times as it may become rancid.)
Turn carrot curls onto a paper towel and pat dry.
Salt to taste.

Cauliflower "Potatoes"

This is a delicious substitute for mashed potatoes.

1 large cauliflower, cut into pieces
¼ cup butter or ¼ cup home-made yogurt

salt, pepper to taste
parsley and paprika garnish

Cook cauliflower until just tender. Drain.
Purée in blender or food processor.
Add butter or yogurt, salt and pepper, and blend thoroughly.
Reheat and serve.
Garnish with parsley and paprika.
The puréed cauliflower may be placed in a baking dish, sprinkled with grated cheddar cheese and heated in the oven until the cheese melts.

Sweet and Sour Lentils

1 cup lentils   *3 tablespoons honey*
2 tablespoons white vinegar   *2 tablespoons butter*

Soak lentils overnight and throw away the water.
Add fresh water to cover lentils and simmer until tender. Drain.
Add remaining ingredients, heat and serve.

MAIN DISHES, POULTRY STUFFING, GRAVY

Baked Bean Casserole

Introduce this recipe when diarrhea has cleared up.

1 lb. dried white beans
1-2 whole onions
meaty bone (ham, beef, etc.)
1 large can tomato juice (48
   fluid ounces)

$^1/_2$ - 1 teaspoon dry
   mustard powder
3 tablespoons vinegar
3-6 tablespoons honey
salt and pepper

Soak beans overnight in cold water. Drain and throw away water.
Rinse beans thoroughly under running water.
Cover with fresh water and simmer at low heat until beans are tender.
This may take over 2 hours. Do not salt beans before boiling; they will not become tender.
Add remaining ingredients and bake in oven at 300°F (150°C) until beans are very soft and tomato juice has thickened.
More tomato juice may have to be added while beans are baking to prevent them from sticking to the pan and burning.
Stir occasionally.
Beans should bake a minimum of 2 hours.
Before serving, cut meat off bone and discard bone.
Serve hot or cold.

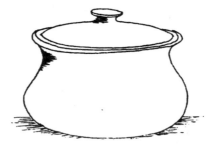

Baked Cottage Cheese

1 cup uncreamed cottage cheese (dry curd)	1 teaspoon honey
1 egg	1 teaspoon butter

Blend all ingredients.

Pour mixture into a greased baking dish and bake at 350°F (180°C) until of firm consistency and slightly browned around the edges (about 15 or 20 minutes).

Chicken Royale

2 lbs. chicken parts	2 whole green onions, including stems, sliced
1 cup sliced or diced carrots	4 cloves fresh garlic
1 cup fresh or frozen cauliflower pieces	1 tablespoon oil
1 whole tomato, diced	½ teaspoon paprika
	salt to taste

Wash and drain chicken parts.

Heat oil, add garlic and green onions and sauté for 2 minutes.

Add chicken and cook for 5 minutes.

Add paprika and tomato, cover and cook for 10 minutes on medium heat.

Add cauliflower, carrots, and salt and cook for another five minutes.

(Recipe courtesy of Zairun and Aleesa Hosein)

Chicken Croquettes

Turkey or cooked ham may be substituted for chicken.

2 cups cooked, boneless, trimmed chicken
2-3 tablespoons almond flour
1 egg
1 small onion, quartered
2-3 tablespoons butter for frying
Season to taste with salt, pepper, herbs, etc.
1 tablespoon chopped parsley (optional)
Sprigs of parsley and lemon wedges for garnish

This recipe may be made in a food processor using the metal blade.
If a processor is not used, finely chop chicken and onion before mixing with other ingredients.

Using the food processor:
Place cubed chicken, onion, egg, and chopped parsley into processor bowl.
Blend until smooth.
Add about half of the almond flour, seasonings, and blend for a few more seconds.
Using your hands to shape the croquettes, determine if mixture is stiff enough to shape. If mixture is not stiff enough, add additional almond flour, a tablespoon at a time, until mixture can be handled easily.
Shape mixture into pancake forms keeping them about 3½" in diameter for easy turning.
Fry in butter over medium heat until golden brown and turn.
Serve hot, garnished with parsley sprigs and lemon wedges.

Poultry Stuffing
(For a large bird)

2 cups dried white beans (navy   1 teaspoon ground sage
   beans)   1 teaspoon ground thyme
1 cup chopped onion   chopped parsley (optional)
1/2 cup chopped celery   salt and pepper to taste

Soak beans overnight and throw away the water.
Cover with fresh water (do not salt before cooking or beans will
be tough) and cook until tender. Drain.
Mix chopped onion, celery, and herbs with beans and mash with
a potato masher.
Season to taste with salt and pepper.
Fill cavity of turkey or chicken with bean mixture and roast.

Ginger-Yogurt Chicken

4 whole chicken breasts   1 teaspoon freshly grated ginger
2 cups homemade yogurt   salt to taste
1/2 cup nut flour   butter for frying chicken

Split each breast down the back into two pieces.
Heat frying pan, add butter and brown the raw chicken. Do not
cook completely.
Salt chicken.
Remove from heat.
Mix yogurt, almond flour, and grated ginger.
Arrange chicken in a single layer in an oven-safe pan.
Spread the yogurt mixture over the surface of each piece of chick-
en, using all of the mixture.
Place, uncovered, in a 325°F (160°C) oven.
Bake ½ hour or until chicken is tender.

(Recipe courtesy of Zairun Hosein)

Gravy

May be used as a thickened gravy for poultry or meat.

Type 1:
While roast is in the oven, boil an onion.
While poultry is in oven, boil an onion together with poultry giblets.
When the meat is done, pour the drippings into a container and skim off fat.
Place cooked onion and skimmed drippings (at least 1 cup) into blender and purée.

Type 2:
For each cup of liquid, add 2 tablespoons of homemade mayonnaise.
Heat gently for about a minute, stirring constantly.

(Recipe courtesy of Roberta Young)

Honey-Garlic Chicken Wings

2 lbs. chicken wings   1 tablespoon lemon juice
1 tablespoon butter   salt and pepper to taste
1/4 cup honey   crushed garlic clove
1 teaspoon grated lemon rind

Place wings in baking dish.
Melt butter and add honey, lemon juice and rind.
Dust wings with salt and pepper.
Pour half of honey mixture over wings and coat evenly.
Bake wings at 350°F (180°C) for 15 minutes.
Add remaining honey mixture.
Continue baking until wings are tender and browned.

Honey-Garlic Spareribs

3 lbs. pork spareribs or ham   2-4 tablespoons crushed fresh
  hocks (unsmoked)   garlic or
1/2 cup honey   4 tablespoons garlic chips
1 cup water   1 teaspoon salt

Parboil pork and remove excess fat if hocks are used.
Mix remaining ingredients and pour over parboiled pork which
has been placed in a large roasting pan or baking dish.
Bake at 375°F (190°C) for at least 1 hour turning and basting at
least twice until the honey begins to caramelize on the meat.

Fish Casserole

1 lb. fresh, frozen, or canned
   fish (halibut, flounder, sole,
   shrimp, lobster, or crab-
   meat)
½ lb. grated cheddar cheese
1 cup homemade yogurt

1 teaspoon dry mustard powder
1 tablespoon chopped parsley
1 tablespoon lemon juice

Poach fresh or frozen fish for a few minutes until cooked through.
Drain, if using canned fish, or cool poached fish, and using fork,
break into bite-size pieces.
Mix remaining ingredients thoroughly and add to fish.
Bake in ovenware at 375°F (190°C) until brown on top. This
should take about 30-40 minutes.
This recipe may also be used as an appetizer. Bake as instructed
and serve in small portions.

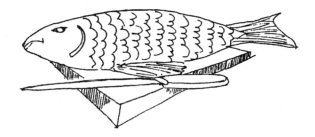

Pizza #1

Crust:

3½ cups coarsely grated,
  unpeeled, zucchini squash†

3 eggs, lightly beaten

⅓ cup almond flour

½ cup grated brick cheese (any
  permissible mild cheese will
  do)

½ cup grated, 100% pure,
  parmesan cheese

1 tablespoon fresh basil leaves,
  minced (dried may be
  substituted but use only
  about
    ¼ teaspoon)

¼ teaspoon salt

†Salt grated zucchini squash with ¼ teaspoon salt and let stand for 15 minutes to draw out excess water. Squeeze zucchini with hands to get rid of as much water as possible.

Mix all ingredients well and spread onto an oiled pizza pan or small cookie sheet. Pat smooth.

Bake for 30 minutes at 325°F (160°C) or until crust is dry and browned.

Brush the top of the crust with oil and broil it under moderate heat for 5 minutes.

Alternative crust recipe: Cheese bread recipe (pg 122) may be used. For a large pizza, use about ⅛ of recipe. Pat down in pizza pan until about ⅓ - ½″ thick. Bake at 350°F until golden brown and proceed by adding filling.

Topping:

½-1 lb. brick cheese, thinly
  sliced

1½ cups tomato sauce (made
  by simmering about 3-4
  cups tomato juice)

a few of the following: mushrooms, olives, strips of green
pepper, crisply fried bacon
pieces, cooked ham slivers,
anchovies, tomato slices, etc.

Layer cheese on baked crust.

Spread generously with thick tomato sauce.

Add your choice of toppings.

Heat pizza in a 350°F (180°C) oven for about 25 minutes until it is very hot and cheese is bubbling.

Serve hot with a tossed salad.

John's Pizza Recipe #2

I have always been a pizza connoisseur, and today I came up with a pizza that I think tastes close to the real thing. It is very simple to make, I hope you like it.

Crust:
½ cup almond flour (add more as necessary for a workable dough consistency)
1 egg

1 teaspoon extra virgin olive oil
¼ teaspoon salt
Italian spices such as oregano and basil to taste

In a bowl mix the above ingredients together and add more flour as needed to form a ball. Oil a pan with olive oil (we use a pizza pan but if you have a non-stick pizza pan, all the better). Add the dough ball pressing down with hands to form the shape of a small pizza crust. Do not worry if it is not as big as the pan.
Preheat the oven to 350°F with the crust in pan (this allows the crust to setup and brown a bit.) By the time the oven heats up, the crust should be crisp and ready for the toppings.

Topping:
Very thin-sliced tomatoes
Havarti cheese
Basil and oregano

Optional:
Italian seasoning may be increased to include others that you like such as garlic, etc.

Drizzle with olive oil and bake for 10 minutes.

(Recipe courtesy of John Higgins and Aggieo)

"Spaghetti" and Sauce

1 lb. ground beef (lean)
1 large can tomato juice (48
*   fluid ounces)*
3-4 fresh tomatoes, if available
1 large onion
1-2 cloves garlic (optional)
1 bay leaf

½-1 teaspoon oregano
1 tablespoon olive oil
salt and pepper to taste
1 spaghetti squash (most large
*   supermarkets can get these*
*   if they don't carry them)*

Sauce:
Chop onion and garlic and brown in oil in a heavy skillet.
Remove onion, set aside, and brown meat in the same pan.
Transfer meat and onion to large pot and add tomato juice, bay leaf, oregano and seasonings.
Simmer to desired thickness; this may take 1 hour or longer.

Spaghetti Squash:
Cut the spaghetti squash in half lengthwise.
Steam on a rack over boiling water in a large covered pan or steamer until just tender. DO NOT overcook as squash can become too soft and watery.
Lift out strings of "spaghetti" from squash with a fork.
Serve smothered in hot spaghetti sauce.
Grated parmesan or romano cheese may be used to top.
The spaghetti sauce may also be used to top boiled white (navy) beans or another type of squash (zucchini, butternut, Hubbard).

Zucchini Noodles

This recipe had its origin in the fact that as much as I like spaghetti squash, I often couldn't find one when I was in the mood for SCD-style "pasta". But I could always find zucchini!

6-8 medium zucchini
  (or 1-2 medium zucchini per person)

Peel zucchinis and remove stem tops.
Using the vegetable peeler, scrape strips off the entire length of each zucchini.
For easier peeling, insert a metal shish kebob skewer down the center, and hold onto the skewer while scraping the "noodles" from the zucchini.
Keep peeling until the entire zucchini is in shreds. Or, if even zucchini seeds are a problem, stop when you reach the seeds and freeze the remaining chunks for vegetable broth.
Pile the zucchini "noodles" on a buttered baking sheet and cook in a preheated 215°F oven for about 25 minutes. The objective of the low temperature is to cook the zucchini while evaporating as much of the excess water as possible.
Serve topped with plain butter and a little salt, or with any of your favorite sauces such as Mock Hollandaise.

(Recipe courtesy of Marilyn L. Alm)

Stuffed Zucchini

6 zucchini squash
1 garlic clove, crushed
1 ½ cups ground beef
1 cup cheddar cheese (or other
   hard cheese), grated
2 eggs slightly beaten

4 tablespoons melted butter
salt and pepper to taste
1 tablespoon chopped fresh
   basil or
   ¼ teaspoon dried basil
   (optional)

Pan fry the ground beef in a little butter until cooked through.
Cut the zucchini squash in half lengthwise and carefully hollow out the flesh to within ¼ inch of the skin.
Set the shells aside.
Chop the zucchini flesh, then press with the back of a wooden spoon to extract as much juice as possible and drain it away.
Set the flesh aside.
Preheat the oven to 400°F (200°C).
Combine the zucchini flesh, garlic, ground beef, basil, cheese, seasoning, eggs and half the melted butter until they are thoroughly blended.
Arrange the zucchini shells skin-side down in a well-greased shallow baking pan.
Stuff with the beef mixture and pour the remaining melted butter over the stuffed squash.
Place dish in oven and bake for 20-30 minutes or until the top is brown and bubbling.
Serve at once.

Zucchini Casserole

Use any amount of the following vegetables; the size of your pan or casserole should be your guide.

zucchini squash, sliced
fresh tomatoes, sliced
onions, sliced
green peppers, sliced (optional)
1 tablespoon salad oil (olive oil
   is best in this recipe) for
   each 4 cups of vegetables

½ cup grated Parmesan cheese
   (optional)
Seasoning: oregano, salt, pepper

Slice raw vegetables and layer in a casserole. A shallow casserole is preferable but any size may be used.

Pour salad oil over vegetables.

Sprinkle seasonings and grated cheese over top.

Add a little water to casserole if there is not sufficient juices from the vegetables. There should be at least ½ inch liquid at the bottom of the casserole when you start baking.

Place in hot oven 400°F (200°C), uncovered, and bake until vegetables are tender.

Stir occasionally so that the top vegetables do not get too brown.

If this recipe is made on top of stove, it turns out to be a vegetable stew and has a completely different consistency.

Zucchini Lasagna

1 ½ lbs. ground beef
2 medium-sized zucchini
  squash, cut lengthwise in ½
  inch slices
2 cups uncreamed cottage
  cheese (dry curd)
1 cup tomato juice

½ cup Colby, brick, or havarti
  cheese, grated or sliced for
  topping.
1 medium-sized onion
1 cup mushrooms, sliced
  (optional)
1 teaspoon oregano
¼ teaspoon ground basil
salt and pepper to taste

Brown meat in a little oil; set aside.

Line baking dish with zucchini slices.

Mix uncreamed cottage cheese with beef and spread over zucchini slices.

Season tomato juice with herbs, salt and pepper and pour over other ingredients

Top with cheese.

Bake at 375°F (190°C) until zucchini squash is tender and cheese blends with other ingredients.

This recipe may be eaten hot as a main course or cold as an appetizer.

Stir-Fried Vegetables with Chicken, Beef, or Pork

cauliflower pieces
broccoli pieces, including the
    stem
celery, sliced
carrots, sliced
zucchini squash, sliced
mushrooms, sliced
tomatoes, quartered

peppers, sliced in strips
onions, sliced
edible-podded peas (optional)
chicken breasts, steamed OR
    sirloin or round steak, semi-
    frozen

The quantity of each ingredient depends on the number of people to be served.

A heavy iron frying pan or a wok should be used.

Sauté in butter, using medium heat, any combination of, or all of, the listed vegetables.

Begin by cooking the vegetables that take longer to tenderize (carrots, cauliflower, broccoli).

After a few minutes, add the rest of the vegetables, except the tomatoes.

Turn heat to simmer, cover pan or wok, and cook until all vegetables are barely tender.

Add tomatoes and cook about 1 minute longer.

Season with salt and pepper.

Add prepared meat or chicken and serve piping hot.

Preparation of meat:

Chicken: Steam until tender. Remove skin and bones. Cut in large chunks. Brown in a separate pan in butter. A little honey may be added to the meat if desired. Set aside until you are ready to combine with vegetables.

Beef: Semi-frozen beef is easy to slice. Slice in thin strips, across grain. Brown pieces of beef in a separate skillet in butter. Set aside until ready to combine with vegetables.

Pork: Use left-over pork roast. Slice in thin strips and set aside until ready to combine with vegetables.

Vegetable Meat Loaf

1½ lbs. ground beef
1 egg
1 medium fresh tomato or ½
*   cup tomato juice*
1 medium onion, cut in pieces

sprig of parsley
1 stalk of celery, cut in pieces
small amount of green pepper
1 carrot, cut in pieces

Place tomato or tomato juice into blender first. Push down on tomato to release juices so that blender blades will turn easily.
Add egg and blend for a few seconds.
Add remaining vegetables and blend until fairly smooth.†
Empty blender contents into bowl and mix well with ground beef.
Season with salt and pepper.
Form mixture into a loaf and place in a shallow pan.
Spread top with homemade quick ketchup (see pg. 92).
Bake at 350°F (180°C) oven for about 1 hour.

†You may have to stop blender and push vegetables down to contact blender blades.

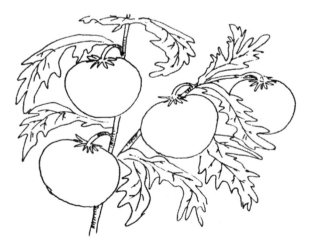

MUFFINS, BREAD, AND PANCAKES

Basic Muffin and Bread Recipe

Nuts suitable for this recipe are walnuts, almonds, pecans, and filberts (hazel nuts). Peanuts should not be used. Although they are usually very expensive, some people prefer unroasted raw cashews. Raw cashews are highly perishable so you must be sure that they have been stored properly. Roasted cashews most often contain starch and are, therefore, not permitted. Your choice of nuts should depend upon price, availability, and personal taste preference. Almonds are usually the least expensive and the choice of most people because of their delicate flavor.

Almonds with skins (brownish in color) are suitable for this recipe although, at the beginning of the diet, blanched almonds (without the fibrous skin) will be less gas-forming. After marked improvement, almonds with skins may be used. Twenty-five pound boxes (or larger) often may be purchased at a discount. If large amounts are bought, they should be kept in the refrigerator or deep freeze to prevent rancidity. In the Appendix, further instructions, regarding ordering nuts in the most inexpensive way, are given.

The nuts must be ground to a fine consistency–a consistency similar to whole wheat flour. If they are overground, they turn into nut butter which may be used but will make the batter a bit more fluid.

It is advisable to grind your own nuts for the first 3-4 weeks on the diet. It is true that ground nuts are available and would be a time saver. It is strongly advised, however, that you grind your own to ensure that the ground nuts are fresh and pure with no added extenders. When you have decided to commit yourself to the diet for a longer period, then the ground nuts can be purchased in large quantities in sealed boxes.

If the nuts are ground in a blender, do not process more than ¾ cup at one time. Grind to the consistency of whole wheat flour stopping the blender occasionally and scraping around the sides with a kitchen knife or spatula.

The food processor grinds nuts satisfactorily: use the steel blade and make sure it runs long enough to grind the nuts to the consistency of whole wheat flour.

The nuts may also be ground in an electric or manual food grinder.

In the recipes that follow, the term "nut flour" will be used interchangeably with the term "ground nuts"; they mean the same thing.

The following ingredients make 16 muffins.
Preheat oven to 375°F (190°C).

2¹⁄₂ cups ground nuts
¹⁄₄ cup melted butter or ¹⁄₄ cup homemade yogurt, or small amount of fruit juice, or pure apple butter (add last and adjust amount depending on the consistency of the batter)

¹⁄₂ cup honey† (more or less as desired)
¹⁄₂ teaspoon baking soda
¹⁄₈ teaspoon salt (optional)
3 eggs (if eggs must be avoided, use puréed fruit to hold ingredients together)

†HONEY: All recipes calling for honey as a sweetener work better if honey is in liquid form. If honey has crystallized, melt over low heat.

Using a blender:
After grinding the nuts in the blender, empty them into a bowl.
Place eggs and honey into blender, and mix thoroughly.
Add the egg mixture to the nuts and blend by hand or with an electric beater.
Add butter or yogurt as needed to bring to a muffin batter consistency.
Blend in baking soda and salt.

Using a food processor:
After grinding nuts, allow the ground nuts to remain in the processor bowl.
Add other ingredients, adding butter or yogurt last according to how much liquid you need to bring the batter to a muffin batter consistency.

Line cupcake tins with paper cupcake liners.
Spoon batter into cupcake tins filling about one-half full.
Bake at 375°F (190°C) for about 15-20 minutes or until muffins spring back when pressed.
It is difficult to bake "light", high muffins without regular flour and the muffins may fall after they have been removed from the oven. This will not affect their taste.

Variations:
1. Add ⅓ cup raisins or currents.
2. Add juice of one orange and some grated orange rind.
3. Add grated orange rind and chopped dried fruit cut into small pieces. About ½ cup of any of these: apricots, sun dried pineapple, apples, pears.
4. Add 1-2 teaspoons of grated orange rind and ½ teaspoon almond flavor.
5. NUT BREAD–Add one more egg (4 altogether) to batter and bake in a well-buttered, 1 quart baking dish.
6. BANANA NUT BREAD–Add one more egg and two mashed extra-ripe bananas to batter.
7. COCONUT-NUT MUFFINS–Substitute dried, unsweetened, grated coconut for part of the nut flour. Do not introduce coconut substitution until diarrhea has cleared up.
8. ELAINE'S FAVORITE VARIATION–After all other ingredients are mixed thoroughly, stir in gently ½-¾ cup fresh or frozen blueberries.

Cheese Bread

This bread can be sliced and used for French toast; dip in beaten egg and fry in butter.
Syrup of hot honey (with a little water added) may be used to top French toast.
Heat oven to 350°F (180°C)

2¹/₂ cups ground blanched almonds (or other allowable nut)
¹/₄ cup softened butter
1 cup bland cheese (brick, Colby, or mild cheddar) cut into very small pieces

1 teaspoon baking soda
¹/₈ teaspoon salt
3 eggs beaten

Mix butter, nut flour, and cheese.
Add eggs, baking soda, and salt.
Pour into a well buttered loaf pan (approx. 4 x 8 inches) and bake until golden brown on top.

Banana Pancakes

1 ripe banana, mashed
1 egg
butter for frying

Beat ingredients together.
Drop on a greased pan and brown over medium heat.
Turn and brown other side.
Serve hot with honey syrup (honey diluted with water and heated)†

†Add maple extract and a little butter to hot honey syrup for a maple syrup substitute.

Deanna's Pancakes with a Twist

4 eggs
2 tablespoons honey
1 teaspoon vanilla
½ teaspoon baking soda
¼ teaspoon salt
1 banana

½ cup uncreamed cottage
    cheese (dry curd)
1 cup almond flour (adjust this
    amount to get pancake bat-
    ter consistency)

Blend all ingredients except almond flour in the food processor until smooth.
Stir in the almond flour.
Pour into a well-buttered frying pan and fry until crispy on the edges.
If syrup is desired, heat up a little honey with a drop of maple flavor.

(Recipe courtesy of Deanna Gold and Katie Fischer)

Deanna's (Midas Gold) Pancakes/Waffles

1 cup almond flour
4 eggs
2 tablespoons honey

1 teaspoon vanilla
¼ teaspoon salt
¼ teaspoon baking soda

Mix together and pour on a greased griddle to make pancakes. Works great in a waffle maker, too!

Herb's Bean Pancakes

Introduce this recipe when diarrhea has cleared up.

*1 cup, soaked, cooked
   and well drained
   white beans*
1 small onion
1 egg

¹/₈ teaspoon baking soda
salt to taste
homemade yogurt as needed

A food processor, blender or electric mixer may be used. If using a blender, place egg in blender first so that blades can turn easily. Place all ingredients in bowl or blender and blend until batter is smooth.
If batter is not a consistency which can be poured easily (as for pancakes), add yogurt, a teaspoon at a time, and blend in well.
Using a well-buttered frying pan, pour batter as you would pancake batter.
Using medium heat, turn pancakes after about 8 – 10 minutes.
Cook an additional 8 minutes on other side.

The above ingredients make 4 medium-sized pancakes.

Do not use beans that have not been drained well as batter will be too watery.

A large batch of beans can be prepared in advance and can be frozen in suitably sized containers.

Lois Lang's Luscious Bread

This bread resembles a moist whole wheat bread. It slices nicely, can be toasted and can be used for grilled sandwiches.

*2¹/₂ cups blanched, ground
    almonds (almond flour)
¹/₄ - ¹/₃ cup melted butter
1 cup dry curd cottage cheese
    (press down as you meas-
    ure*)*

*1 teaspoon baking soda
¹/₄ teaspoon salt
3 eggs*

Preheat oven to 350°F (180°C)
Place eggs, melted butter, dry curd cottage cheese, baking soda, and salt in food processor using metal blade. Process until the mixture is thick and resembles butter in texture.
Add almond flour and process until mixed thoroughly. If the stiffness of the mixture stops the processor, remove the dough with wet hands and knead by hand until almond flour is thoroughly mixed into other ingredients.
Grease a loaf pan (about 4" x 8") generously with butter and coat bottom with ground almond flour.
Using wet hands, shape dough into a loaf shape and press into greased pan.
Bake at 350°-375°F for about 1 hour until lightly browned on top. There will be a crack on the top of the loaf. Check by inserting a metal kitchen knife; it will come out clean when bread is done. Remove from oven and run a metal spatula around the sides of the pan pressing gently against the loaf to loosen it at the corners and bottom of pan.
Remove bread by inverting the pan onto a cake rack. Allow to cool thoroughly before you cut it. Don't cut it while it is piping hot. It needs to firm up its texture.

Variations:
1. Add 1 tablespoon caraway seeds with the flour and you will get bread that resembles rye bread.
2. Add about ½ cup raisins and/or other dried fruit as a last step when you are kneading it into a loaf shape and you will have a tea loaf.
(Recipe courtesy of Lois Lang)
*If you are unable to find the dry cottage cheese, use one cup of the drained homemade yogurt (Cream cheese recipe–pg. 158).

Zucchini Muffins

3 cups grated zucchini
3 eggs, beaten
3 cups nut flour
$^1/_3$ cup melted butter

$^1/_2$ - $^2/_3$ cup liquid honey (use less, if desired)
2 teaspoons cinnamon
1 teaspoon baking soda
$^1/_2$ teaspoon salt

Mix almond flour, melted butter, honey, and zucchini.
Add beaten eggs, cinnamon, salt, and baking soda. Mix well.
Bake in muffin tins, lined with papers, at 350°F (180°C) for
about 20 minutes or until done.

Sandwich Rolls

This recipe makes 12 rolls – perfect for cheeseburgers or turkey
sandwiches with bacon, lettuce, and tomato.

1 cup uncreamed cottage cheese (dry curd)
¼ cup melted butter
¼ cup honey

1 tsp. baking soda
3 eggs
2½ cups almond flour

The secret in making rolls that don't flatten (although flat tastes
good too), is to add the eggs after the first four ingredients. For
fluffy batter, do not let the processor run too long after the
addition of the eggs.

Mix first four ingredients briefly in the food processor and beat
until it is fluffy – like whipped cream. Add eggs and beat briefly.
Remove from processor and add almond flour. Stir in thoroughly
with a mixing spoon or spatula. Put large tablespoons of batter on
a greased baking sheet and run a wet hand or spoon over each
roll. Bake at 350°F (180°C) for about 15 minutes.

(Recipe courtesy of Steve Diehl)

CAKES

Banana Cake

3 cups nut flour
3 eggs, beaten
1/4 cup melted butter
1/2 -2/3 cup honey

1 teaspoon baking soda
2 mashed bananas
(extra ripe)

Mix all ingredients.
Pour into a buttered baking pan.
Bake at 350°F (180°C) until top springs back when touched (about 40 minutes).

Carrot Cake

1½ cups nut flour
1½ cups finely shredded carrots
¾ cup honey
½ cup raisins
½ cup walnuts (optional)

1 teaspoon baking soda
½ cup butter
2 eggs
1 teaspoon cinnamon
pinch salt
1 teaspoon vanilla

Add honey and eggs to softened butter and blend.
Blend in nut flour, soda, salt, cinnamon, and vanilla.
Add carrots, raisins, and nuts.
Bake at 350°F (180°C), 45-60 minutes.
This cake has a tendency to overflow; therefore, use a large baking pan. A one-quart (1 liter) loaf pan lined with greased waxed paper is satisfactory.
This recipe may be used as a carrot pudding by decreasing the amount of almond flour.

Cheese Cake

The cheese cake filling may be made without a crust but for special occasions, when you want a crust, line the bottom of a small loaf pan with Almond honey crisp recipe (see page 130), keeping it as thin as possible.
Bake crust and cool thoroughly.

Filling:

3 eggs
⅓ cup honey
½ cup homemade yogurt or cream cheese made from yogurt (see pg. 155)

2 cups uncreamed cottage cheese (dry curd)
2 teaspoons vanilla extract
1-2 teaspoons grated lemon rind

Place all ingredients in blender or food processor (metal blade) putting eggs in first so that blender blades will turn freely.
Blend until smooth stopping, if necessary, every 15 seconds to push ingredients down, scraping the sides of the container at the same time with a spatula.
Pour into loaf pan with or without crust.
If desired, place drained, unsweetened canned pineapple slices on top of filling.
Bake in oven at 350°F (180°C) for about 30 minutes or until edges are brown.
Cool and refrigerate.

Date Loaf

3 eggs
½ cup honey
½ cup melted butter
½ cup homemade yogurt
½ teaspoon baking soda
3 cups pecan or almond flour

1 teaspoon salt
½ pound pitted, chopped dates
  (California dates only)
pecan or walnut pieces

Preheat oven to 325°F (160°C).
Mix together all ingredients, reserving pecan or walnut pieces for top.
Pour batter into a well greased and floured (with nut flour) loaf pan.
Decorate top with nut pieces.
Bake until knife placed in center comes out clean – about 45 minutes.

(Recipe courtesy of Lois Lang)

Nut Torte

1½ cups blanched almonds or pecans
½ cup honey
8 egg whites

Grind nuts, ¾ cups at a time, in blender.
Return ground nuts to blender, add honey, and blend well.
In a large mixing bowl, beat egg whites until stiff.
Very gradually fold honey-nut mixture into egg whites.
Pour into three greased layer cake pans.
Bake at 350°F (180°C) for about 35 minutes or until a kitchen knife comes out clean.
Cool. Fill between layers with custard filling (page 137) or honey frosting (page 134).

COOKIES

Almond-Honey Crisps

This recipe may also be used to make a pie crust. Line pie plate with parchment paper to prevent sticking.

1 cup whole almonds
1/4 cup butter
1/3 – 1/2 cup honey

2 teaspoons vanilla (unsweet-
ened)

Process nuts in a blender for only a few seconds until nuts are coarsely chopped. Do not overchop or you will get a flour-like texture which is not suitable for this recipe.
Place chopped almonds in a bowl and set aside.
Put butter, honey, and vanilla in blender, pushing ingredients down to bottom of container before turning blender on.
Process for about 30 seconds until ingredients are whipped.
Transfer mixture to bowl containing chopped nuts and blend thoroughly with a spatula.
Spread in a shallow cake pan and bake at 375°F (190°C) until golden brown.
Cut into squares while still warm.

Cheese Cookies

1/2 cup dry curd cottage cheese
1 egg white

1 teaspoon honey
2 teaspoons nut flour

Mix ingredients.
Drop on greased cookie sheet.
Bake in 325°F (160°C) oven until brown.

Date-Filled Cookies

4 cups nut flour
1/3 cup butter, melted
1/4 teaspoon baking soda

1/4 teaspoon salt
1/2 cup honey

Mix all ingredients well.
Roll into small balls.
Place on a greased cookie sheet and press balls into flat cookies with the back of a buttered teaspoon.
Bake at 300°F (150°C) until golden brown.
Remove from pan and cool.

Filling:
1 lb. pitted dates
(California dates only)
1/3 cup water

Put dates and water in a covered oven-safe saucepan and bake in the oven until soft. This should take about 15 minutes in a 350°F (180°C) oven. This date mixture can be cooked on top of stove but it has a tendency to scorch if not stirred constantly.
Stir occasionally while in oven.
Heat in oven until thick.
Cool.
Spread date filling between two cookies.

Peanut Butter Brownies

1 cup peanut butter, no additives (almond butter may be substituted)
1/2 cup honey

1/2 teaspoon baking soda
1 egg

Mix all ingredients thoroughly, and pour into a well-buttered eight inch square baking dish. Bake at 350°F (180°C) for about 25-30 minutes. Remove from oven when nicely browned.
Cool slightly and turn out of pan. Cut into brownie squares.

Peanut Butter Cookies

When first trying these cookies, it is a good idea to restrict your intake to two per day. They are so delicious, people have been known to eat a whole batch in just two or three days, which can cause a flare-up, especially early on in the diet.

½ cup butter	*1 cup nut flour*
1 cup peanut butter, no additives	*2 eggs*
	¼ teaspoon baking soda
½ cup honey	*1 teaspoon vanilla*

Cream butter until soft.
Add peanut butter and mix thoroughly.
Add remaining ingredients.
Drop on greased cookie sheet and bake in 325°F (160°C) oven for 10 minutes.

Monster Cookies

5 cups nut flour	*½ cup melted butter*
1 cup raisins	*1 cup honey*
1 cup walnut pieces	*2 eggs, beaten*
1 cup flaked unsweetened coconut	*1 teaspoon baking soda*
	⅛ teaspoon salt

Mix all ingredients.
Drop by large tablespoonfuls onto greased cookie sheet.
Press flat with a buttered fork. If fork is greased, it will not stick.
Bake at 325°F (160°C) until golden brown (15-20 minutes).

Pumpkin Cookies

3 cups nut flour

1 cup mashed, cooked, drained
  pumpkin or fresh or frozen
  winter squash such as
  butternut or acorn. Do not
  use canned pumpkin.
  Summer squash such as zucchini is too watery for this
  recipe.

½ cup butter

1 egg

¾ cup honey

1 teaspoon baking soda

¼ teaspoon salt

¼ teaspoon cinnamon

¼ teaspoon nutmeg

1 teaspoon vanilla

1 cup raisins

Mix dry ingredients and raisins. Set aside.
Mix egg, butter, honey and vanilla in blender.
Add pumpkin or squash to egg mixture and blend thoroughly.
Add wet ingredients to the dry mixture.
Drop by rounded teaspoonfuls 2 inches apart on lightly greased
cookie sheet.
Bake 15 minutes at 375°F (190°C) until lightly browned.
Transfer to wire rack to cool.
Makes about 4 dozen cookies.

(Recipe courtesy of Nancy Ferguson)

FROSTINGS

Cream Cheese Frosting

1½ cups dry curd cottage cheese or
*   drained homemade yogurt*
honey to sweeten

Place a little liquid honey in blender.
Gradually add dry curd cottage cheese or drained yogurt.
Blend until smooth.
It may be necessary to stop blender occasionally and press cheese
down so that the blender blades can make contact.
Use as a frosting on carrot cake or banana cake.

Honey Frosting

1 cup honey
1 egg white, beaten
1 teaspoon vanilla

Boil the honey until a drop forms a firm ball in cold water.
Add gradually to beaten egg white.
Whip until stiff and add vanilla.
This frosting is marshmallow-like and remains spreadable for
hours.
Use as a frosting for cakes; this frosting is especially good on the
nut torte.

Honey Cream Whipped Topping

2 cups French Cream (see recipe page 158)
1 teaspoon vanilla
½ cup honey

Combine all ingredients and whip to stiff peaks.

(Recipe courtesy of David J. Couture)

DESSERTS

Apple Custard Pie

4 or 5 baking apples
1 tablespoon lemon juice
$^1/_2$ cup honey
3 eggs
$^3/_4$ cup homemade yogurt or
    homemade French Cream
    (see page 158)

$^1/_4$ cup apple cider
$^1/_4$ teaspoon nutmeg
2-3 tablespoons chopped
    almonds or walnuts

Core and cut the apples into eighths.
Toss them in lemon juice which has been mixed with honey.
Arrange the apple slices round side down in a pie plate with a circle around the outer edge and another circle inside that, filling in the center.
Bake in oven at 400°F (200°C) for 20 minutes.
Beat the eggs slightly, stir in yogurt or French Cream, apple cider and nutmeg.
Pour egg mixture over the apples and continue baking another 10 minutes.
Sprinkle the top with the chopped nuts and bake 10 minutes longer or until the top is golden and the center firm.
Cool on a rack before cutting.

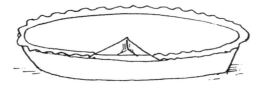

Applesassies

½ cup butter	*1 cup nut flour*
½ cup honey	*¼ teaspoon baking soda*
2 eggs, lightly beaten	*1 cup walnuts, chopped*
⅔ cup homemade applesauce	*¾ cup raisins*

Melt butter in a double boiler.
Sir in honey, eggs, and applesauce.
Mix baking soda with nut flour and stir into butter mixture.
Stir in raisins and walnuts, saving a few walnut pieces for topping.
Turn into a greased 9 inch square pan.
Sprinkle with the reserved walnuts.
Bake at 350°F (180°C) for about 30 minutes.
Cool in pan and serve topped with honey-sweetened whipped uncreamed cottage cheese or French Cream.

(Recipe courtesy of Anne Haas Hall)

Baked Honey Apple Slices

½ cup honey	*2 teaspoons butter*
juice of 1 lemon	*½ teaspoon cinnamon*
3 large cooking apples	

Mix honey and lemon juice in shallow baking dish or pie pan.
Peel and core apples.
Cut apples in quarters, then slices.
Place in honey-juice mixture, coating well.
Dot with butter.
Bake in a moderate oven, 350°F (180°C) for about 30-40 minutes or until tender.
Baste with pan liquid twice during baking.
Can be topped with same cheese mixture as Applesassies (above).

Custard

2 eggs
1 cup uncreamed cottage cheese
 (dry curd)
2 teaspoons vanilla extract

8 teaspoons honey
dash of nutmeg
pinch of salt

Beat uncreamed cottage cheese and eggs in blender of food processor until very smooth.
Add honey, vanilla and salt. Beat thoroughly.
Pour mixture into custard cups.
Sprinkle nutmeg on top of each cup.
Place custard cups in a pan half filled with water.
Bake at 350°F (180°C) for about 20 minutes. Increase heat to 375°F (190°C) for another ten minutes or until browned on top.

Honey Glazed Whole Apples

4 medium cooking apples
1 cup water
1 cup honey

½ cup uncreamed cottage
 cheese (dry curd) which has
 been blended until smooth
 with a little homemade
 yogurt.

Pare and core apples.
Bring water and honey to a boil in a deep saucepan.
Slowly cook 2 apples at a time in a covered pan in the syrup until apples are tender, turning apples occasionally.
Remove to dessert dishes.
Boil syrup until thick.
Cool syrup slightly and pour over apples.
Serve warm or chilled, topped with blended uncreamed cottage cheese or French Cream.

Honey-Walnut Baked Apples

large apples for baking	*1 tablespoon honey for each*
raisins	*apple*
walnut pieces	*cinnamon*

Choose a variety of apple that bakes well such as McIntosh, Spy, Ida Red.

Core the apples with a sharp knife leaving them whole.

Arrange apples in a baking dish.

Mix together enough raisins (or currants) and walnuts with honey to fill the cored-out apples.

Add cinnamon to this mixture according to taste.

Fill the apples with honey mixture.

Bake at 350°F (180°C) until apples are tender when poked with a fork (about 1 hour).

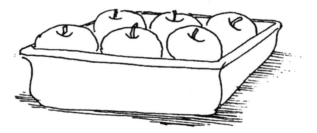

Ice Cream

1 mashed banana or ¹/₂ cup puréed unsweetened peaches, pineapple, or strawberries

1-2 cups homemade yogurt honey or saccharin for sweetening according to taste
¹/₈ teaspoon salt

Blend ingredients well.

Place in paper cups or popsicle molds and freeze.

For real ice cream texture, this mixture may be placed in an ice cream maker.

Adjust amounts of ingredients depending upon the volume of your machine.

If you have an ice cream maker which calls for crushed ice, you can avoid having to crush the ice by doing the following:

In the space in which the crushed ice is to be placed, pour 1 cup of cold water.

Measure about 2 cups of ordinary salt and make layers of ice cubes, alternating with salt, until the space is filled. Use all the salt by the time you reach the top.

It is wise to have available plenty of ice cubes; save up the equivalent of about 6 trays before starting.

Pour another cup of cold water around the top of the cubes. Start up the motor of the ice cream maker; it should be done in less than an hour.

Variation: Add 1 or 2 raw eggs to the mixture for a creamier texture.

Instant Blender Ice Cream

2 cups homemade yogurt
1 quart frozen fruit
    (strawberries, raspberries, sliced peaches, blueberries)
Note: Do not thaw fruit!
honey to sweeten

Place ½ cup yogurt in blender.
Gradually add frozen fruit and the remaining yogurt alternately.
Add honey to taste.
Blend until thick.
Store in freezer until ready to eat.
This ice cream is thick and smooth and should be eaten soon after making.
If it is refrozen, it will crystallize.

Variation: Freeze yogurt in ice cube tray and in blender mix the frozen yogurt cubes with pineapple juice or other juice (or a mixture of both juices). Use about 6 yogurt ice cubes and ½ cup juice adding small amounts of juice to obtain a thick consistency.

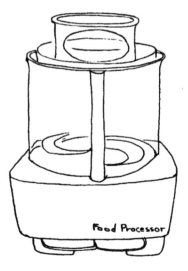

Food Processor

White Bean Ice Cream

*2 cups cooked white beans
   (well drained)
3 cups homemade yogurt
1 cup honey*

*4 large eggs
¼ teaspoon salt
2 tablespoons vanilla*

Beat eggs, honey, and salt together in top of double boiler.
Place over boiling water and cook until thick, stirring constantly.
Set aside while you prepare the rest of the ingredients.
Place ¼ cup of yogurt in bottom of blender.
Add beans, one cup at a time, and process until very smooth.
Add ¾ cup of yogurt and blend well.
Pour into a very large bowl, add remaining 2 cups of yogurt.
With electric beater running, add custard mixture slowly beating
constantly.
Add vanilla and mix well.
Place in freezer and as the mixture freezes at the sides of the con-
tainer, mix with unfrozen part. This should be repeated a few
times until the ice cream is completely frozen.
This mixture can be placed in a commercial ice cream maker of
any type instead of freezing in the freezer.

Variations:
1. When ice cream is beginning to thicken, stir in ½ cup apple
    butter.
2. Mashed or puréed banana, peaches, pineapple, strawberries
    can be folded in as mixture freezes.

(Recipe courtesy of Lois Lang)

Pineapple Cheese Dessert

1 envelope unflavored gelatin
$1/8$ cup cold water
2 beaten egg yolks
2 stiffly beaten egg whites
$1/2$ cup unsweetened crushed
*   pineapple*

1 teaspoon lemon juice
$1/2$ teaspoon lemon rind, grated
$1/2$ cup uncreamed cottage
*   cheese (dry curd)*
$1/4$ cup honey
dash of salt

Soften gelatin in cold water.
Combine egg yolks, pineapple, lemon juice, lemon rind, honey, and salt. Cook over hot water until thick.
Add gelatin and stir until dissolved.
Remove from heat, add cheese.
Chill until set.
Fold in stiffly beaten egg whites.
Spoon into individual molds and return to refrigerator.

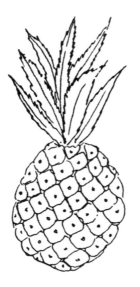

Lemon Soufflé

1 tablespoon melted butter	3 eggs
½ cup honey	juice of 1 lemon
¼ cup almond flour	1 cup homemade yogurt

Separate egg whites and beat until stiff.
Beat egg yolks.
Add butter, honey, almond flour, and lemon juice to egg yolks and mix well.
Stir in yogurt.
Fold egg whites into mixture.
Pour into greased soufflé dish or deep baking dish.
Set in a pan of water and bake at 350°F (180°C) for about 30 minutes.
Soufflé is done when an inserted knife comes out clean.

Raspberry Mousse

2 cups homemade yogurt	4 cups fresh raspberries (2 cups puréed)
2 envelopes unflavored gelatin	½ cup honey
3 eggs separated	

In the top of a double boiler, blend egg yolks, puréed raspberries, honey, and yogurt.
Heat over boiling water, stirring constantly until hot.
Place gelatin in ½ cup cold water for a few minutes to soften.
When raspberry mixture is hot, add softened gelatin and mix thoroughly.
Remove from heat and chill until mixture starts to set.
Whip egg whites to stiff peaks and fold into raspberry mixture.
Chill until firm and serve with remaining raspberries arranged around the mousse.

(Recipe courtesy of David J. Couture)
(Submitted by Barbara Scheuer)

Raspberry Mousse Angel Pie

Meringue Crust:

3 large egg whites, at room
   temperature
1/8 teaspoon salt

1/4 cup honey
1/2 teaspoon vanilla extract

Preheat oven to 275° F.
Lightly oil a 9″ pie plate and set aside.
In a large mixing bowl, combine egg whites and salt.
Beat until soft peaks form.
Add half of the honey and beat for 30 seconds.
Gradually beat in the remaining honey.
Add vanilla and beat until all the honey is dissolved and the meringue is stiff and shiny.
Spread the meringue over the bottom and sides of the oiled pie plate.
Using the back of a spoon, spread some meringue up to the rim, forming a decorative edge.
Or, using a piping bag fitted with a star tip, pipe the meringue into the pie plate.
Bake for about 1 hour and 15 minutes or until firm and crisp.
Cool on a wire rack. (The meringue crust can be prepared ahead and stored, covered, in an airtight container for up to one week.)

Raspberry Mousse Filling;

1 package (12 oz.) frozen,
   unsweetened raspberries,
   thawed
   (3 cups)
2 tablespoons (2 envelopes) unflavored gelatin
1/4 cup orange juice or apple
   cider

1 1/2 tablespoons fresh lemon
   juice
1/2 cup honey
1/4 teaspoon salt
1/2 teaspoon vanilla extract
1 1/2 cups homemade yogurt
Mint sprigs for garnish

Set aside a few raspberries in refrigerator for garnish.
In a food processor or blender, purée the remaining raspberries and their juice.
If desired, strain the pureed raspberries through a fine strainer to remove seeds.

Set aside.

In a small saucepan, sprinkle gelatin over $\frac{1}{2}$ cup cold water.

Let stand for about 3 minutes to soften.

Stir in orange juice or apple cider and lemon juice.

Heat over low heat stirring for 1-3 minutes or until gelatin is dissolved.

Add the raspberry puree, honey and salt.

Increase heat to medium and cook, stirring for 3-4 minutes or until honey dissolves.

Remove from heat and add vanilla extract.

Pour the raspberry mixture into a heatproof bowl and set over a larger pan of ice water.

Stir gently for 10-20 minutes or until the mixture thickens to the consistency of raw egg whites.

Whisk in yogurt.

Pour into cooled meringue crust.

Cover loosely with plastic and refrigerate until set for at least 3 hours or for up to 8 hours.

Garnish with reserved raspberries and mint sprigs.

Serves 10

(Recipe courtesy of Carol Clark and adapted from Susan G. Purdy's recipe published in Eating Well magazine, May/June 1992.

Submitted by Barbara Scheuer)

Strawberry Mousse

2 cups homemade yogurt
2 envelopes unflavored gelatin
3 eggs, separated
½ cup sliced strawberries
   (optional)

6 tablespoons puréed strawberries
½ cup honey (more or less as
   desired)

Beat egg yolks thoroughly with a fork, and pour into the top of a double boiler or saucepan.
Blend ½ cup of yogurt and strawberry purée with the egg yolks.
If using saucepan, place mixture over low heat and stir until hot.
If using double boiler, place mixture over boiling water and stir until hot.
Add honey and stir thoroughly.
Place contents of two envelopes of gelatin in ½ cup cold water for a few minutes to soften.
Add softened gelatin to hot mixture, stirring constantly for a few minutes. Remove from heat.
Add enough yogurt to increase volume of mixture to 3-4 cups. Mix thoroughly.

Note: For each envelope of gelatin, do not exceed two cups of mixture. Place in refrigerator until mixture begins to set. This should take about 1 hour.
Beat egg whites until stiff.
Fold sliced strawberries into beaten egg whites.
Fold strawberry-egg white mixture into gelatin mixture.
Return to refrigerator until gelatinized completely.

Variations: Other fruits may be used: canned, unsweetened crushed pineapple, puréed apricots or peaches.
(Recipe courtesy of Nancy Marcellus)

Pumpkin Pie

The Almond honey crisp recipe (see pg. 130) may be used as a crust or this recipe may be made without a crust and eaten as a custard or pudding.

Filling:
  3 eggs, beaten
  1 cup homemade yogurt or
    uncreamed cottage cheese
    (dry curd) puréed
  ½ cup honey
  2 cups of prepared squash or
    pumpkin (canned not per-
    mitted)†

Spices:
2 teaspoons cinnamon,
  1 teaspoon nutmeg,
  ½ teaspoon ground cloves.
  Spices may be varied according to preference.

All ingredients should be mixed thoroughly. This may be done in a large mixing bowl using a beater, in a blender, or in a food processor. Because of the large volume, it is advised that only part of the ingredients be placed in the processor or blender at one time to avoid overflow.
Pour into a large pie pan or two smaller ones.
Bake at 375°F (190°C) or until a knife comes out clean.
May be served warm or cold.

†To prepare squash or pumpkin:
Use winter squash (hubbard, acorn, or butternut).
Remove seeds and steam, boil, or bake until tender.
Scoop out insides discarding skin. Drain.
A large pumpkin may be baked or cooked until tender in the same way as the squash.
Place pumpkin in a bowl and let stand to drain.
Scoop out insides.
Freeze what is not used.

SWEET TREATS, JAM

Candied Nuts

*1 lb. nuts (almonds, walnuts,
    pecans, hazelnuts) shelled
If hazelnuts are used, rub in
    towel to remove skins.*

*2 egg whites
½-¾ cup honey depending
    upon desired sweetness
¼ cup melted butter
pinch of salt
pinch of cinnamon*

Place nuts on large shallow pan and toast in oven at 300°F
(150°C) for 10 minutes.
Cool.
Beat egg whites with salt until peaks form.
Gradually add honey and continue beating until honey and egg
whites are thoroughly mixed.
Fold in nuts and cinnamon.
Coat the large shallow pan with melted butter.
Spread nut and egg white mixture over buttered pan.
Bake in oven at 300°F (150°C) for 30 minutes turning nuts every
10 minutes until butter disappears.
Let cool in pan.
Cut or break into bite-size pieces and store in covered container.

(Recipe courtesy of Judy Newman)

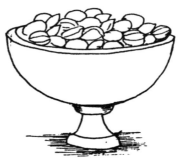

Granola Chews

$^1/_4$ - $^1/_3$ *cup butter*
$^1/_2$ *cup honey*
$^1/_2$ *cup raisins*
$^1/_2$ *cup unsweetened, grated coconut*

1 cup coarsely chopped nuts (almonds, pecans, or walnuts)
$^1/_2$ *teaspoon salt*

In a saucepan, stir butter and honey over low heat until melted and blended.
Remove from heat and add remaining ingredients, combining well.
Spread mixture in an ungreased square 8 inch baking pan.
Bake at 350°F (180°C) for about 25 minutes until set.
Cool, cut in squares.

Quick, Uncooked Coconut Ball Candy

1 cup liquid honey
½ cup unsweetened, grated coconut
½ cup chopped nuts

Blend ingredients and roll into balls using buttered hands (to prevent mixture from sticking to hands).
Balls may be rolled in chopped nuts.

Vanilla Candy

½ cup water
1 lb. honey (about 2 cups)
1 teaspoon vinegar

1 teaspoon vanilla extract
   (more, if desired)
2 tablespoons butter
crushed nuts (optional)

Heat honey with vinegar and water in a large pot.
Allow to boil gently until a soft ball forms when dropped into cold water.
Remove from heat and add vanilla extract and butter.
Mix thoroughly with a spoon.
If nuts are to be used, add nuts to honey mixture.
Pour into a flat, buttered *metal* pan and cool.
Place in freezer until hard. Only then can it be cracked into small - bite-size pieces.
Remove pan from freezer; place it on a board. Using a clean screw driver as a wedge, crack candy in several places by hitting screw driver handle with a hammer.
Return to freezer to store.
This recipe may be used for making nut logs as follows:
Use 1-2 cups pecan or walnut halves.
When honey mixture is ready to remove from heat, add nuts, butter, and vanilla and mix thoroughly.
Cool nut-honey mixture and spoon onto wax paper (doubled in thickness).
Roll into logs and refrigerate.
Slice as needed.

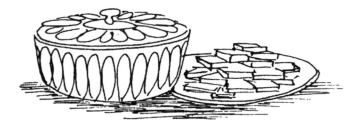

Lolly Pops

Have available small clean sticks; may be purchased in hardware store. Follow the recipe for vanilla candy by heating honey, vinegar and water in a large pot.

Allow to boil gently until a *firm* ball forms when dropped into cold water.

Remove from heat and add vanilla extract but *no butter*.

Place sticks about 4 inches apart on a greased cookie sheet and pour approximately 2 tablespoons of hot mixture at the top of each stick allowing mixture to cover about ½ inch of the top of the stick.

When the candy has hardened, remove lolly pops and wrap separately.

Variation: Flavorings such as anise or cinnamon may be added with the vanilla.

Becky's Magic Toffee

This recipe is a variation of the vanilla candy recipe.

½ cup water	1 tablespoon vanilla extract
1 lb. honey	1 tablespoon baking soda
1 teaspoon vinegar	

Heat honey, vinegar, and water in a large pot.

Allow to boil gently until a *firm* ball forms when dropped into cold water.

Remove from heat, place pot in sink, add vanilla extract and baking soda.

Stir briskly but only until baking soda is thoroughly blended in and toffee mixture foams up.

When the foaming begins to subside, pour into a well-buttered pan and cool.

When candy is *firm* enough, it may be cut into bite size pieces using kitchen shears or cracked with a blunt instrument.

Variation: When candy has cooled enough to handle, it can be pulled like taffy and then cut into pieces. Children will enjoy the taffy pull.

(Recipe courtesy of Becky Smith)

JAMS

Jams can be made with many different fruits: strawberries, raspberries, peaches, apricots, black currants, or a combination of these.

Commercial pectin is not to be used.

To make jam, add ½ cup honey for each quart of prepared fruit.

Add the smallest amount of water possible to simmer the jam and keep it from sticking and burning at the beginning of cooking.

Stir until ingredients are well blended, then simmer, stirring occasionally to prevent sticking.

As jam becomes thicker, stir more often to prevent scorching.

The jam is done when it becomes thick and forms droplets on the edge of a spoon.

The cooking process should take from 1–1 ½ hours depending on the amount of water to be evaporated.

The jam may not be as thick as ordinary jam. Do not risk scorching it to get it thicker.

Place small amounts in clean containers and freeze. Thaw as needed.

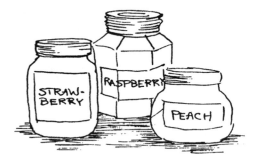

BEVERAGES

Almond Milk

1½ cups ground almonds
3 cups water
1 tablespoon honey (optional)

Combine and blend for several minutes in a blender. Drain through a colander lined with a cheese cloth

Milk Shakes

For 1 cup:
 ½ cup homemade yogurt
 ½ cup fresh or frozen fruit, such as strawberries, peaches, raspberries, bananas, blueberries.†

Place yogurt in blender and then add fruit.
Sweeten to taste with a little honey or saccharin.
Blend until thick and creamy.

†If fresh fruit is used, add a few ice cubes to chill drink.

Fruit Juice Spritzer
(Replacement for pop)

Combine fruit juice† with Perrier water or club soda and ice to make a nutritious, "fizzy" drink.

†Naturally sweetened juices suitable for this recipe are apple cider, orange, grapefruit, pineapple, and grape.

Party Punch†

1 quart unsweetened pineapple juice
about 1 quart of orange juice, not from concentrate

Mix juices in punch bowl, add ice cubes.
Float fruit slices or berries on top.

†Keep a bowl of punch available, especially in warm weather, to avoid the temptation of beverages that are not permitted. Make sure punch bowl is sturdy.

Piña Colada

unsweetened pineapple juice
ice cubes

Fill blender no more than half full with unsweetened pineapple juice. Add no more than 4 or 5 ice cubes.†
Run blender for about 45 seconds until drink is frothy and creamy.
Serve at once.

†If sherbet is desired, rather than a drink, add about 10 ice cubes.

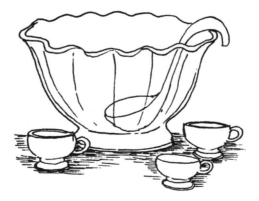

MILK PREPARATIONS AND INFANT FORMULA

YOGURT

Yogurt is one of the oldest foods known to man. Wherever people milked cows, goats, mares, sheep, or camels, a product similar to yogurt was eaten. Kefir, Kumiss, fermented acidophilus milk, and Bulgarian milk are all similar to yogurt, differing only in the kinds of microbes introduced into the milk.

If milk is left unrefrigerated in a warm environment, many types of microbes (bacteria and yeast) in the air, as well as some remaining in the milk, even after Pasteurization, start multiplying and using the milk sugar, lactose, as a source of energy. The result is soured milk which often has a bitter, unpleasant taste and consistency. In making yogurt, this process is controlled by getting rid of the mixture of microbes and introducing only those which produce the tart and tasty product you desire.

You may use powdered, skim, 2%, or whole milk. If you use powdered milk, add only the amount of powder which you would use to make regular fluid milk. **Do not** add additional milk powder to fluid milk in order to get a thicker yogurt or more protein as you will not get a "true" yogurt and it **will be detrimental** to those on the Specific Carbohydrate Diet.

Whole milk makes a very tasty yogurt but if you are eliminating fat for a particular reason, you may use low fat milk. If you do, you must be careful while heating as it scorches more readily than whole milk.

INSTRUCTIONS
1. Bring one quart (or liter) milk to the simmer stage and remove from heat. Stir often to prevent scorching and sticking to the bottom of the pan.
2. Cover and cool until it has reached room temperature (20-25°C / 64-77°F or below; may be placed in refrigerator to hasten cooling). It is very important that you allow the temperature to drop sufficiently or you will kill the bacterial culture you are now ready to introduce.
3. Remove about one-half cup cooled milk and make a paste with one-quarter cup of good quality commercial yogurt. The

commercial yogurt you use should be unflavored and unsweetened. Buy one containing only milk or milk solids and bacterial culture. Recommended cultures are *Lactobacillus bulgaricus, L. acidophilus,* and *S. thermophilus.* Avoid yogurts and starters containing *bifidus.* It is usually unnecessary to buy yogurt culture separately since commercial yogurt is very satisfactory to use as a "starter". If you find it impossible to buy commercial yogurt which contains only milk and bacterial culture, then you are advised to buy yogurt culture ("starter") separately. After removing what is needed, return the container of commercial yogurt to the coldest part of the refrigerator for use as a starter in the next batch of homemade yogurt.

Saving some yogurt from a previous batch of homemade yogurt to start a new batch is not as satisfactory as using commercial yogurt as a "starter" each time. Manufacturers of commercial yogurt make every effort to use "lively" bacterial strains and extremely large numbers of bacteria in the manufacturing process. The conditions of home refrigeration most often do not promote the survival of yogurt bacteria to the same degree as the conditions maintained by the commercial yogurt producers. Homemade yogurt, made by using some of the the last batch as a "starter", often fails to solidify (coagulate) properly due to insufficient quantities of live bacteria.

4. Mix the paste with the remainder of the cooled milk and stir thoroughly.

5. Pour milk into any appropriately-sized container, cover, and let stand **for at least 24 hours** at 100°-110°F (38-43°C). (If you forget to remove it after 24 hours, and the fermentation goes on longer, all the better.) Under no circumstances should the fermentation time be decreased to less than 24 hours. This fermentation time should supersede any other instructions which may accompany a commercial yogurt maker.

The source of heat used during the 24-hour fermentation is critical. It is very important to get the temperature correct at 100°-110°F (38-43°C) before you proceed with the fermentation. Too high a temperature will kill the bacterial culture and will prevent the proper "digestion" (conversion) of the lactose. Too low a temperature will prevent activation of bacterial enzymes and will result in incomplete "digestion" of the lactose.

A thermos-type yogurt maker may not be satisfactory for this long fermentation period as the hot water surrounding the thermos will not stay warm. The electric commercial yogurt makers control the temperature perfectly but the amount of yogurt that can be made at one time is limited. An ideal source of heat is a large electric warming tray. If it has a temperature-regulating dial, use a thermometer to set the dial properly. A mouth thermometer is adequate. If the warming tray does not have a dial to control the temperature, cover the surface of the tray with a thickness of metal (such as a metal cake rack) or **fire-resistant material** (such as a teflon-treated ironing board cover) and allow the tray to remain on for about five minutes before placing the thermometer on the surface to determine the temperature. If too warm, use a thicker piece of metal or material. By using the large surface of the electric warming tray, a gallon of yogurt can be made at one time in two, plastic or ceramic, half-gallon containers.

Some people use their ovens; the pilot in a gas oven usually keeps the temperature in the oven within the correct range. If using the oven of an electric stove, change the oven light to a 60-watt bulb. Turning on the oven light (with a 60-watt bulb) should create enough warmth to make yogurt; always check the temperature with a thermometer first. Sometimes the oven door must be propped ajar with a little stick to achieve the correct temperature range.

Caution: Upon completion of yogurt fermentation, replace regular oven bulb.

6. Allow the yogurt to remain on the heat for a minimum of 24 hours to ensure that all lactose is completely "digested". Remove from heat gently and refrigerate.

While this yogurt may not be as thick as commercial yogurt, it will be a **true** yogurt since virtually all of the lactose has been digested by the bacterial culture and further lactose digestion will not be required by intestinal cells.

NOTE

See INTERNET SECTION for mail order yogurt makers and cultures.

Cream Cheese

1   Line a colander with a clean cloth (a dish towel is satisfactory).
2. Place colander on a bowl.
3. Pour chilled yogurt into lined colander and allow to drain for about 6-8 hours (need not be refrigerated while draining).
4. Lift cloth by two opposite ends, place on flat surface, and with a spatula, scrape "cream cheese" off and refrigerate. It will be quite tart; a little liquid honey may be worked in with a spatula to sweeten.

French Cream

*2 cups cream
    (table cream, half-and-half,
    or heavy cream)*

*½ cup commercial yogurt
    (see yogurt recipe for type to
    use as starter)*

Bring cream to simmer stage stirring often as it heats.
Cool cream and follow recipe for homemade yogurt.
Allow cream to ferment for 24-48 hours.
Refrigerate.
For a creamy rich ice cream, use in ice cream recipe instead of yogurt or use part yogurt and part French cream. May also be used as a topping for desserts.

INFANT FORMULA - DISACCHARIDE FREE

This formula may be used for short periods of time until the physician can prescribe a formula which contains no disaccharides. Some commercial formulas, recommended for diarrhea, contain considerable amounts of corn syrup (containing maltose and iso-maltose). As a result, some babies with severe diarrhea do not recover when they are used[1]. Check newer formulations as they appear on the commercial market to ensure they are disaccharide-free.

The following formula (about 2 cups) contains approximately 90 mg calcium, 175 mg phosphorous, 72 mg potassium, 0.40 mg iron, 17 gm protein, 0.3 gm fat, and 2.7 gm carbohydrate.

Babies one year and younger need approximately 500-700 mg calcium per day. An additional source of calcium would, therefore, be necessary if this formula is used more than a few days. Please discuss this with your physician.

The following ingredients should be used and enough water added to bring the total up to about 2 cups (17 fluid oz or 500 ml).

3 tablespoons uncreamed cottage cheese (dry curd) (1.2 oz or 33 gm)
1 tablespoon unrefined safflower oil (0.7 fluid oz or 19 ml)

It is preferable to purchase the oil already bottled. Health food stores and some large supermarkets usually carry this item. Please read the label carefully and make sure that there is no BHT or BHA added. Addition of vitamin E, beta carotene, or vitamin A is all right.

2 tablespoons pasteurized honey (0.9 fluid oz or 25 ml)

Prior to the preparation of the formula, place the honey and approximately 1 cup of the water in a pressure cooker and heat keeping the honey-water mixture under pressure for 10 minutes. This is to sterilize the honey and kill any microorganisms which cannot be killed by ordinary heat.

Place the dry curds in a blender with the oil.

Blend until very smooth.

Slowly add the honey-water mixture and blend until smooth.

Bring total up to approximately 2 cups (17 fluid oz or 500 ml) with water.

Place in a nursing bottle and make the hole in the nipple slightly larger.

This recipe may be doubled or tripled depending upon how much the baby needs. Keep the unused portions refrigerated and covered. Use within 24 hours after preparation.

The formula contains the following:

Total protein, mainly casein	1.1%
Total carbohydrate	5.0%
Total fat	3.8%

These proportions are comparable to breast milk with the exception of the carbohydrate. Breast milk contains 2% more carbohydrate. However, the formula does not contain all the vitamins and minerals that are needed daily by the baby. The formula may be tried, with your doctor's concurrence, for a limited period for constipation or diarrhea. When the condition is alleviated, return to the normal formula.

Addendum

THE MOM AND DAD BRIGADE

This section is dedicated to the memory of my husband, Herbert Adrian Gottschall, who held me up when I could no longer stand. Our daughter's words, written on Father's Day, 1993, thirty years after we "knew" she was cured, inspired me to add this section to the book.

Dear Dad,

I remember you running along School Lane, hanging on to the back of my two-wheeler, never letting go as I extracted promises by the second that you won't – and, finally I do it! I remember your driving me to horseback riding lessons every Sunday, your stopping at the gas station so I could throw up from fright, but your still urging me to go on and just adoring those lessons.

I remember your calm strength through terrible times when Mom could not muster one more ounce of courage through my illness but you had me convinced that I would get better. And I did!

I remember a lot more too because you were a wonderful Dad. You taught me how to cherish my kids because you did us.

Forty-five years ago my own child was diagnosed as having an incurable disease, ulcerative colitis. This book is a testament of our family's journey from hopelessness, helplessness, and isolation to a return of not only health for my child, but a desire to prevent needless suffering of other families.

Will the feeling of, "I must talk to someone who understands," ever leave me? During the years of her illness, each time I heard of someone else with inflammatory bowel problems, the strong urge to communicate overpowered me. I would call strangers anywhere in the world just to talk and seek some measure of understanding and consolation.

It has become apparent to me that, as important as scientific information has been to bring about recovery in our children, the support of spouses, friends, and others is not only beneficial but also essential. Those who have battled the storm of bowel disease with their own loved ones can give confidence and a large measure of reassurance to those just entering the fray.

The Addendum of this book is a record of some of the inspiring and compassionate support offered by parents to others as they embark on the Specific Carbohydrate commitment. Most of this help was given via the Listserv* on the Internet. These parents have allowed me to include their words in this supplement to *Breaking the Vicious Cycle*.

* A group of over 600 people supporting each other on the Internet. Information pertinent to the SCD (Specific Carbohydrate Diet) is shared. The Listserv was started by Rachel Turet after her recovery from ulcerative colitis, which has been replaced by:
http://health.groups.yahoo.com/group/BTVC-SCD/ and
http://health.groups.yahoo.com/group/BTVC-SCD-Advanced/

From Cindy

Hi! Three months ago my 7-year-old started having stomach pains from bad gas and bloating (his stomach gets really hard and distended). We started with a GI specialist who put him through a ton of tests that have shown nothing so far. A month into this, he also started moving his head from side to side and bending at the waist. He didn't do this all the time, but eating and exercise started the movements. The gas seems to be a trigger for everything going wacky. He had a hard time holding his head up after eating a bagel and was put in the hospital for three days, undergoing a ton of neurological tests that all came back negative.

I read about *Breaking the Vicious Cycle* at Amazon.com and ordered it. At this time we are all devastated here as we are dealing with something that no one has even diagnosed as of yet. I really think this started with gastrointestinal problems and everything is related. When I read this book I started crying uncontrollably because I know I have to do it and it seems so daunting. But I know I have to if the diet can take away the unbelievable gas and bloating and, maybe, some of the neurological symptoms.

I want to know if there is anyone else out there who has experienced bending and tilting of the head (my son tells me this makes his stomach feel better) and also if there are any yummy recipes a 7-year old would like.

This is going to be tough for him and all of us. My husband and I are doing it too, for the support we can give him. I know we have to do this, but it is so scary to a Mom who isn't a good cook and never aspired to be. Any words of encouragement will be so much appreciated.
Thanks, Cindy.

The following emails followed within minutes of Cindy's request.

From Lisa D.

Reading your letter brought back all the feelings we went through when our son became ill. It was such a horrible time and we just didn't know what to do. It was like every black cloud ever created was hovering over us. During the worst of our son's illness, I don't believe I ever slept. I spent countless hours sitting in my living room praying, crying, wondering, and feeling overwhelmed and defeated. I wondered how much longer my son could endure the ravages of this disease and what it was doing to his body (at this time he had not as yet been diagnosed with ulcerative colitis). When he was finally diagnosed, there was a feeling of elation for us for, at least, we knew what he had. It had a name! There was something we could do about it. However, no doctor, at this time, told us that drugs were a short term answer. After seven years of going through a series of drugs each time a drug failed to work, we found this diet.

It was as if God opened up the Heavens! We now know that if my son stays with the diet sufficiently long, he will be well. I wondered at the time if I could manage it and now, after a year, I can tell you things become easier.

All I can say is, give the diet a try, give yourself time, and don't beat yourself up over mistakes because you will make them. We all have. In the end it will give your child a wonderful gift and you will have given yourself a whole new sense of purpose. Please know that we will try to be as helpful as we can and do not be afraid to ask questions and voice your fears. Lisa D.

From Brenda:

Cindy, I know you can do it. I have Crohn's and an ileostomy now. I've had Crohn's for 16 years and an ileostomy for 3 years. My son was showing signs of bowel problems so he was colonoscoped and subjected to other tests, which showed nothing. I put him on SCD (I'm on it too) and everything cleared up.

He had a lot of gas pains in his stomach and his chest wall. He also had trouble keeping his feet still. In his own words at 10 years old, after putting him on the diet for about 2 weeks, he told me his feet didn't want to move anymore. That winter he excelled at school and also in indoor soccer as he was much more focused. After a while, his friends, our family and the teacher became very accustomed to his eating habits and it wasn't a big deal at all. In fact the neighborhood kids sure like those peanut butter cookies.

As a Mom I can see that you will be surprised to find what you can do when your own kids are involved. I'm a single parent and my son is now 13. 1 do not want to see anybody go through that emergency surgery I went through to have my ileostomy. Hope this helps, Brenda

From Keri Klein:

Cindy, you can do it! I didn't experience head bending, but gas and distension were symptoms of mine before I started on this diet. The gas is gone. The distension is much improved.

People on the Listserv will respond and here are some ideas to try, after you follow the introductory diet in Breaking the Vicious Cycle. Remember, try one new food at a time at the beginning. Smoothies made from homemade yogurt, ripe banana, honey, strawberries. Peanut butter and honey spread on peeled apples. Cheese chips: grate cheddar cheese. Melt small piles in skillet until crispy and flip and cook the other side, then cool until hard.

There are so many great recipes for cakes and desserts in Breaking the Vicious Cycle and Lucy's Cookbook. And don't forget you can make him frozen yogurt treats by pouring smoothies into popsicle molds and freezing. Good luck, Keri

From Katie:

Hi, Cindy. A lot of people believe that intestinal problems cause a lot of other weird problems. I am sure that this diet is worth a try. I never thought I could follow it, as I was a total pizza and junk food addict. I was also deathly ill from Crohn's and have three little kids, five years old and under, so I had to do it. Now six months later, I am miraculously in remission and feeling wonderful for the first time in 25 years (I am now 35).

I love this diet. I wouldn't have believed that before. There are so many wonderful substitutes for most foods. The nut flour baking is wonderful and is extremely healthy. The most important thing is to never let your son get hungry. You know how hard it is to resist temptation when you are hungry. Always keep plenty of snacks available, and here are some, which we find especially good:

Peanut butter cake, monster cookies, cinnamon cookies from Lucy's Cookbook, coconut cookies, macaroons, frozen yogurt, cashew peanut butter, the muffins from BTVC, frozen juice pops.

I am sure some of the moms will write you with their favorites. Oh, one more: cheese fries made out of fried Monterey jack cheese sticks. It does seem hard at first, but it really seems easy after a while. It just becomes a habit. Good luck. Katie

And another email of encouragement from Pam Williams

Your anxiety and love for your son came through loud and clear in your posting on the SCD list. The diet looks daunting, we know, especially for someone who doesn't love cooking. As another uninspired cook, let me share how SCD can change the way you think about food.

The hardest part is getting started. Many SCDers said to themselves, "I'll try it for a month and see how it goes." If your son is like hundreds of people on this list, he'll start to feel better within that month. You'll start to appreciate that what goes in his mouth contributes to his well being and health, and that diet is a natural, ancient way to nurture the people you love and positively affect their well being.

Before SCD, I would go completely blank in a supermarket when faced with all the options and absolutely no inspiration to cook them. On the SCD, I went from eating whatever was easy and handy to feeling all proud and nurturing when my yogurt came out soft and snugly. Food changes from a chore to a healthy, natural tool to get back some control in a situation that seems out of control and out of your hands.

With love, Pam.

And from Donna Bauchner, Brett's Mom

Just to re-introduce myself. I'm the Mother of a fifteen year-old, Brett, who has been on the SCD for about ten months. Brett has Crohn's, but thanks to SCD has been living life like any other teenager: school, going out with friends, playing baseball, lifting weights, marching in the school band, and, generally, having a wonderful life.

Brett decided to share his success on the SCD with others and has posted information about SCD on various websites for inflammatory bowel disease sufferers. The response that he has received has been wonderful. So far, he has directed several people to the Listserv. Of course Brett did hear from one skeptic who attacked Brett's endorsement of SCD with a vengeance! Brett didn't let the doubter get to him and yesterday felt so good when he was able to talk about diet and Crohn's with two distraught parents whose teenagers are very ill.

They sounded as crazed as I was when Brett was first diagnosed, and they seemed eager to investigate the SCD further. I am so proud of my son and just wanted to let you know how important it is to try the diet for your son. Donna

And from Martha

I'm Jonathan's mom. I've been swamped with activity lately and haven't been able to write but I want you to know that I am thinking of you.

Jonathan is 10 and was diagnosed with Crohn's disease two years ago. We started the diet about then on our naturopathic doctor's advice. I know that the beginning may seem rough, but now, one year later, my SCD (Specific Carbohydrate Diet) family of five is all thriving and I am cooking with ease. The cup can be viewed as half full; think of the frontier women without supermarkets, electricity and appliances (that sounds like my Grandma's life with a lot more children to cook for).

Several people on the list wrote to me with suggestions on how to get through the first few parties. You can bring substitute food for your son such as homemade pizza, legal cake, etc. At this point, however, my son simply accepts that he will not be eating all that other stuff without any expressed negative emotion. You will get there too, once you witness how the diet makes everyone feel better.
Good luck, you are on the right path. Martha

From Lisa Ercolano:

Your post about how much Danny is suffering brought tears to my eyes! My daughter, Olivia, is 11 (and has Crohn's disease) and she, too, had lost weight due to the disease and its symptoms.

But good news, though. She has gained 4-1/2 pounds in the three-plus weeks that she has been eating the Specific Carbohydrate Diet. There is no question that it may seem difficult at first. We had not yet realized how easy it is to get the few substituted ingredients. However, within a week, we had stocked our fridge with all kinds of fruits and vegetables; I bought legal canned fruits and made "cocktails" of the different kinds, and finally got going with the homemade yogurt.

I know your son is not as old as my daughter, so it is probably a little more difficult to explain to him the fact that eating only healthy foods will help him get well. But if you do the hard thing – to get rid of anything in your cupboards that is not SCD, he will eat the goodies you make, he really will. He will also quickly learn that he feels better when he eats these things so he will want to eat more. I have found that eating this diet with Olivia helps her to accept it. It is how the rest of us show support for her and belief in the diet.

I know from first hand experience how painful it is to see one's child wasting away. But all I can do is reassure you that this way of eating WORKS.

Hang in there. Eat SCD yourself. Let Danny bake and cook with you if he feels up to it. Your boy will be bouncing back in no time is my guess. It wouldn't hurt to do something nice for yourself like a hot bubble bath and good book when he is in bed. You are under a lot of stress.

From Patty

I just had to chime in here. My daughter, Tabitha, just turned 7, has Crohn's disease. She has been suffering from this monstrous thing since she was at least 4 years old. She would tell you the diet is definitely worth it. In fact, she was just telling me earlier, "my tummy doesn't hurt any more since I have been on the diet."

Before we found the diet, my precious baby only weighed 32 pounds. That is very small for, at that time, she was 6 years old. She had a mean fistula in her rectum. I watched with horror as my sweet Tabitha bled into the toilet time after time. Just thinking about the torture of it all gives me a very queasy feeling. My heart ached for her, as she was unable to play and at times too weak to even get out of bed. I started her on the diet about a month ago, and she is very glad that I did. I have complete control over what she eats because I homeschool her. I keep a food and weight diary and record her symptoms daily. After all that we have been through, I want to give the diet an honest chance and keep a careful record to eliminate all doubts.

A week or two before we started the diet, Tabitha's SED rate (test for inflammation) was 78. Two weeks after starting the diet, it was 5. She is symptom free, weighs 44 pounds and is bursting at the seams with energy. She plays every day now. A simple thing such as playing is a big thing to me and to her.

I hope my email helps in some way to keep you focused. You may hit some rough patches from time to time, but I think you can stay on the road.

And from Krysia to the author

Dear Mrs. Gottschall,

My name is Krysia Morin and I am eleven years old. I am writing to tell you that without your helpful book I would not be the healthy girl that I am today.

I started having bad stomachaches when I was six and as the years went by the pain worsened until I could not sleep at night. We used a scale from one to ten to gauge the pain with ten being the worst. Sometimes the pain reached eight on the scale. My Mom took me to the doctor several times but all they did was take more tests. One doctor even said, "Wait until she is stunted before doing anything."

Mom kept going to the library and finally found your book and we decided to try it out. Within a week the pain went down to three and sometimes one. Within six months, the pain had totally stopped. I have been on the diet for three years and only when I eat forbidden foods will I get a stomach ache.

I want to thank you again for all the work and research that you put into your book and I will never forget what you have done for me.

Yours truly, Krysia Morin

Isaiah's Story

Isaiah is a 12 year old boy with regressive Autism. He was born perfectly normal, and actually progressed ahead of schedule. A series of ear infections, oral antibiotics, immunizations, and an exposure to the wild virus strain of chicken pox caused Isaiah to suffer a loss of language, eye contact, joint attention, behavioral self-modulation, and the general ability to verbally communicate his needs, problems, and pain. He developed a severe and persistent gastrointestinal overgrowth of yeast, alternating constipation and diarrhea, food allergies, seasonal allergies, autistic ente-rocolitis, and lymphoid hyperplasia. It was so painfully debilitating that it caused him to cry and scream, as he tried to find physically comfortable positions. It also caused him to miss many days of school.

Isaiah followed a strict casein and gluten free diet for the past six years, with variable and minor improvement. He continued to battle chronic yeast overgrowth, clostridia, alternating diarrhea and constipation, abdominal pain, gas, and bloating. He failed to acquire social and language skills, to the degree it seemed he should. In retrospect, his tantrums, mood changes, and behavioral outbursts, were all essentially related to his state of bowel function and dis-comfort.

In a practice of treating well over 100 children with diag-noses of Autism Spectrum Disorders, I must say that despite rigorous implementation of the casein-free and gluten-free diet (or free from any identified IgG allergens), as well as informed supplementation, I have not seen children improve to the extent and in the fashion one would antici-pate. These children cannot implant normal flora, or eradi-cate clostridia or yeast. Despite nearly heroic interventions to correct these problems, and heal the gut, we see continu-ing deficiencies in nutrients, fatty acids, and amino acids, as well as on-going bowel problems.

Since starting the Specific Carbohydrate Diet six months ago, Isaiah has demonstrated impressive progress. He has had a normal stool every day since the third day on the diet. On the one occasion that he was exposed to birthday cake and ice cream, he developed diarrhea for two days, and cried the entire time. When he resumed the SCD, the diar-rhea and crying stopped, and have not returned. Isaiah has made significant, rapid progress in developing more lan-guage skills. His sentence structure has become more com-plex, he utilizes appropriate pronouns, and engages in spontaneous conversation. He has developed an interest in football, forsaking more juvenile interests, such as "Thomas the Tank Engine". He has become a champion speller. He has been included in the full-day, sixth-grade classroom, with supports. Last year, he spent 50% of his school-time alone with an individual teacher, because he could not stop crying, and performing almost-constant obsessive-compulsive routines. He missed over 50 days of school last year due to severe abdominal pain, crying, pacing, and screaming. Learning is difficult, at best, under those circumstances.

With love, respect, and gratitude, Pamela J. Ferro

Further details regarding Isaiah's Story may be found on the website: www.breakingtheviciouscycle.info.

* *

Some emails ask why something is considered an illegal food on the diet. Although the scientific ground rules are given for practically every food eliminated, often individuals want more detailed reasons. To answer every one of these questions would be impossible. The inclusion or elimination of certain foods is based on the clinical findings of Dr. Sidney Valentine Haas's work as reported to the author in the 1970's, as well as many years of research on the chemical structures of certain molecules – work done by the author.

An outstanding email was sent in by Daphne to one of the "questioning" correspondents.

It sounds as though you are having trouble with your friend's adherence to the diet. Can you help him understand that trying to analyze the contents of every item on SCD is a zero sum game? The nature of organic molecules is extremely complex. A glucose molecule alone contains 24 atoms in a complex three-dimensional structure, and any given starch can contain thousands of simple sugars attached in a huge variety of configurations. Then there is the interaction of carbohydrates with heat, time, and other components of food. And there are so many factors in how our bodies interact with foods – our bacterial ecosystems (1000s of different micro-organisms), the many enzymes that break down foods, our microvilli, our cellular absorption. Most popular nutrition books break nutrition into three categories: carbohydrate, protein, and fat. But in reality, it is far more complex.

The Specific Carbohydrate Diet should be considered evidence-based medicine. We follow it because it works for many people. Period! If we try to tweak it to our hopes and wishes, you will get nowhere but very confused.

Nutrition is still in the dark ages – about where pure chemistry was 150 years ago. The importance of vitamins was only recognized in the middle part of the twentieth century. Compound that with the massive influence of the food industry on science and medicine, and the fact that the chemical composition of foods is changing rapidly due to agritech, etc. And consider the difficulty of conducting clinical trials in nutrition because there are so many factors for which to control. And consider the fact that each scientist can only focus on one tiny piece of a huge puzzle.

The Specific Carbohydrate Diet is a beacon of light in a black hole of misinformation as far as I am concerned. But until the time that teams of researchers and millions of dollar can be put into it, no one can answer your every question about "why".

INTERNET SITES

The advice on the websites listed below conforms to the Specific Carbohydrate Diet.

(1) www.breakingtheviciouscycle.info
This is the official website for *Breaking the Vicious Cycle*. This site gives details to those wishing to know more about the Specific Carbohydrate Diet (SCD) including a beginner's guide, knowledge base and valuable insights into the SCD.

(2) www.scdiet.org – The SCD Library
This is an archive of testimonials, history of SCD, Frequently-Asked Questions, physician resources, and many recipes. This site also links to other sites which are established in Danish, Dutch, Finnish, German, and Spanish languages and additional North American sites in English.

(3) www.scdiet.com
Book and video marketing relating to the Specific Carbohydrate Diet. Some videos are recordings of lectures given by Elaine Gottschall at conferences and/or TV interviews; biographies of the scientists who developed the SCD, as well as the complete first chapter of *Breaking the Vicious Cycle*.

(4) www.scdkitchen.com
Mail order kitchen shop where appliances (yogurt makers, ice cream makers), yogurt cultures, and other necessary ingredients for the SCD may be ordered.

(5) www.pecanbread.com
An excellent, well-maintained site offering support for parents of children on the SCD for intestinal problems and/or autism.

(6) www.healingcrow.com
Discussion on health issues with much information on the Specific Carbohydrate Diet. There is a special section called SCD Wisdom with detailed answers to questions by the author of *Breaking the Vicious Cycle*.

(7) www.scdrecipe.com
Additional recipes for the Specific Carbohydrate Diet as well as interesting and humorous comments by site managers.

(8) www.uclbs.org
A resource, especially for those living in the Toronto, Ontario area containing some excellent recipes.

(9) www.regimeGS.com
A French language website with information on the SCD and other topics relating to the diet.

(10) www.giprohealth.com
Especially helpful to those looking for information related to autism and the SCD. It offers recommendations if dairy cannot be tolerated and discusses vitamins, minerals and probiotics.

(11) www.gottschallcenter.com
Based on the SCD, the Gottschall Autism Center will partner with families to provide children and adults with optimal health interventions, support services, educational enrichment and employment opportunities.

(12) http://health.groups.yahoo.com/group/BTVC-SCD/
This is the main discussion group for people following the SCD. It is a friendly group of dedicated SCDers who provide help to those geting started on the SCD, trouble-shooting for those already on the diet, and general support.

(13) http://health.groups.yahoo.com/group/BTVC-SCD-Advanced/
This Group is for individuals who have been following the diet for at least one year.

GLOSSARY

Carbohydrates	various types of sugar, starch, and dietary fibers
Digestion	(1) the process of reducing large food molecules into simpler compounds and, thereby, making it possible for them to be absorbed from the digestive tract into the bloodstream (2) splitting food molecules
Disaccharides	sugars composed of two parts (two molecules) chemically linked and which require digestion before they can be absorbed into the bloodstream
Disaccharidases	a group of enzymes embedded within the membranes of the intestinal absorptive cells. These enzymes (lactase, sucrase, maltase, and isomaltase) digest (split) the double sugars lactose, sucrose, maltose, and isomaltose respectively
Enteropathy	an intestinal disease
Enzymes	chemical compounds, made by cells, which are responsible for chemical reactions carried on by those cells
Fermentation	the chemical breakdown of carbohydrates (sugars, starch, and fiber) by intestinal microbes resulting in the production of hydrogen gas, carbon dioxide gas, and various other products such as lactic acid, acetic acid and alcohol.
Fructose *(levulose)*	(1) a monosaccharide sugar found in honey and fruits (2) one of the monosaccharide sugars released, along with glucose, when sucrose is digested (3) a "predigested" sugar
Flora	various bacteria, yeast, and other microscopic forms of life in the intestinal contents
Galactose	a monosaccharide sugar released, along with glucose, when the milk sugar, lactose, is digested
Glucose *(dextrose)*	(1) a single sugar (see monosaccharides) found in sources such as fruits and honey (2) a single sugar released, along with fructose, when sucrose is digested

(3) a single sugar released, along with galactose, when lactose is digested

(4) the single sugars released when maltose and isomaltose are digested

(5) the type of sugar making up the starch molecule; starch is a chain of glucose molecules

Lactase   an enzyme embedded within the membranes of intestinal cells (within the microvilli) which digests (splits) lactose into glucose and galactose

Lactose   (1) milk sugar

(2) a disaccharide sugar composed of one part glucose and one part galactose chemically linked

Lumen   interior space of intestine

Maltase   an enzyme embedded within the membranes of intestinal cells (within the microvilli) which digests (splits) maltose into two molecules of glucose

Isomaltase   an enzyme embedded within the membranes of intestinal cells (within the microvilli) which digests (splits) isomaltose into two molecules of glucose

Maltose   a disaccharide sugar composed of two molecules of glucose chemically linked; most of the maltose found in the intestinal tract is derived from starch which has undergone partial digestion

Isomaltose   a disaccharide sugar composed of two molecules of glucose chemically linked differently than maltose; most of the isomaltose found in the intestinal tract is derived from starch which has undergone partial digestion

Molecule   a substance containing two or more atoms. Example: water is a molecule which contains two atoms of hydrogen and one atom of oxygen (H_2O).

Monosaccharides   (1) single sugars including glucose, fructose, and galactose which require no further digestion in order to be absorbed into the bloodstream

(2) "predigested" sugars

Mucosa   the lining of the intestinal tract which is formed by the

(intestinal)   intestinal cells and which comes in contact with the contents of the intestinal tract

Peristalsis   involuntary waves of muscular contraction and relaxation which propel the contents of the intestine forward

Polysaccharides   a class of carbohydrates consisting of many chemically linked sugar molecules; starch is the most familiar example

Putrefaction	the chemical breakdown of proteins by intestinal microbes resulting in the formation of ammonia and other substances

Refined Carbohydrate

a carbohydrate such as cornstarch or white sugar which has been separated from substances with which it is normally associated in the natural or whole state. Refined carbohydrates usually have their calories left intact but have lost most, if not all, of the fiber, vitamins, and minerals found in the whole foods from which they have been extracted.

Starch	(1) a long chain of glucose molecules chemically linked to each other (2) one of the carbohydrates found throughout the plant kingdom; grains and potatoes contain large amounts of starch (3) a polysaccharide
Sucrose	(1) a disaccharide sugar composed of one part glucose and one part fructose chemically linked (2) ordinary table sugar extracted from sugar cane or sugar beets
Sucrase	an enzyme embedded within the membranes of the intestinal cells (within the microvilli) which digests (splits) sucrose into glucose and fructose
Sugars	chemical compounds of varying sweetness which include fructose, glucose, isomaltose, lactose, maltose, and sucrose
Villi	finger-like projections (forming hills and valleys) which normally make up the absorptive surface of the small intestine; they become flattened in various conditions
Microvilli	finger-like projections normally present on individual intestinal absorptive cells; normally, digestive enzymes are embedded within microvilli but, in many conditions, microvilli disappear along with their digestive enzymes
Vitamins	substances present in small amounts in natural foodstuffs (or supplements) which are essential for cellular function and the lack of which in the diet results in disease. The cells, with minor exceptions, cannot make vitamins.

APPENDIX

CHEESES

Permitted cheeses are those which contain virtually no lactose. In order for a cheese to be free of lactose, the manufacturing process must include separation and removal of the whey (containing most of the lactose) from the curd as well as a "curing" of the remaining lactose by the addition of a bacterial culture.

Cheeses Permitted	Cheeses Not Permitted
Use those in italics freely; the others occasionally	Cottage Cheese (regular)
Asiago	Cream
Blue	Feta
Brick	Gjetost
Brie	Mozzarella (Pizza Cheese)
Camembert	Neufchatel
Cheddar, mild, medium, (sharp cheddar – occasionally)	Primost
Colby	Ricotta
Edam	Processed cheese slices or spreads
Gorgonzola	Pre-packaged shredded cheese
Gouda	
Gruyere	
Havarti	
Limburger	
Monterey (Jack)	
Muenster	
Parmesan (if already grated, check to ensure that there are no added milk solids)	
Port du Salut	
Roquefort	
Romano	
Stilton	
Swiss	
Uncreamed cottage cheese (dry curd)	

Amount of Sucrose Commonly Added to Foods

Food category	Average percent by weight
Baked goods, baking mixes	11.42
Breakfast cereals	26.71
Grain products, such as pasta or rice dishes	1.43
Processed cheeses	24.56
Frozen dairy desserts	9.31
Processed fruits, juices and drinks	12.58
Fruit ices, water ices	12.38
Processed meat products	2.87
Processed vegetables, juices	13.25
Condiments, relishes, salt substitutes	26.82
Soft candies	44.74
Jams, jellies, sweet spreads	32.72
Sweet sauces, toppings, syrups	30.96
Gelatin, puddings, fillings	19.11
Processed nut products	8.14
Gravies, sauces	5.66
Hard candy	49.98
Chewing gum	42.30
Granulated sugar	97.92
Instant coffee and tea	12.60
Baby Products	
Cereals	2.55
Formulas	4.76
Processed fruit	12.25
Meat products	0.44
Poultry products	0.58
Processed vegetables	2.89
Puddings	12.09
Soups, soup mixes	0.36

Sources for Vitamin Supplements

It is important to find vitamin supplements which contain no sugar, starch, wheat, soy, whey, or yeast. A yeast-based supplement is not permissible while on this diet. This eliminates brewer's yeast and most natural B-complex vitamins.

People living near large cities or towns should be able to contact companies or individuals who can supply them with information about the fillers and binders used in various vitamin preparations. The information given on pages 66 and 67 of this book gives the reader some idea as to what strengths of each vitamin are appropriate.

Although it is more convenient to obtain vitamins locally, often this is not possible. In these cases, the author suggests that you contact Freeda Vitamins. Their Quin B Strong (with Vitamin C and zinc) is the recommended B-Complex vitamin for people on the Specific Carbohydrate Diet. Ask for the SCD-formulated Quin B Strong. Cut the tablets in quarters or halves depending upon the amount needed. In Chapter 9, amounts are suggested for members of the B-Complex vitamin family which are believed to be suitable for the average adult or child who has a malabsorption problem. Since these vitamins are not scored for cutting, it will take a little patience to cut them evenly. Do not be too concerned if you find you cannot be exact.

To contact Freeda Vitamins:
47-25 34th Street, Long Island City, New York, 11101
Toll-free:1-800-777-3737
Web site: www.freedavitamins.com
Email: FreedaVits@aol.com

There are many companies making good quality B-Complex vitamins, but it is beyond the scope of this book to investigate them. If you prefer dealing with a company in your vicinity, it is your responsibility to contact them and ask about the forbidden binders and fillers such as starch, lactose, whey powder, and sucrose which are often combined with vitamin compounds. If you take vitamins with starch and other forbidden carbohydrates, you lose the benefit of the diet.

SOURCES FOR GROUND AND WHOLE NUTS

For the first three weeks that you try the diet, it is advisable that you buy nuts by the pound (or kilo) and grind them yourself. People in or near large cities, with a little effort, can locate a source of nuts at a reasonable price. You have a choice of health food stores, bulk food stores, wholesale/retail outlets (listed in phone book), and specialty companies which supply food items for those on special diets. Bakeries use nuts in their baked goods; ask at the bakery about their supplier.

When you are convinced, after the first 2-4 weeks, that the diet is helping you, then it is more economical to order the ground (minced) blanched almonds or ground pecans in a large quantity. There should be considerable saving when you order a 25 lb. or 35 lb. box. It is important to keep the ground nuts under refrigeration or in a freezer to prevent rancidity. The Internet section lists sources for the ground nuts.

Mail Order SCD Kitchen Shop

Lucy's Kitchen Shop supplies quality yogurt makers, yogurt culture, blanched almond flour, ice cream makers, food dehydrators, and a Specific Carbohydrate cookbook.

The blanched almond flour from Lucy's Kitchen Shop is whole almond flour. Some nut flours can be a byproduct (what is left over after the oils are pressed out). Byproduct nut flour should not be used by those on the Specific Carbohydrate Diet.

With several years of strict adherence to the Specific Carbohydrate Diet, Lucy can offer assistance with getting you started.

Lucy's Kitchen Shop

www.lucyskitchenshop.com
or
www.scdkitchen.com

888-484-2126 toll free
360-647-2279 outside the U.S.

All recipes are grain, sugar, and virtually lactose free.

"Last night we had Chicken Italiano for the first time and it was wonderful! We also like the Cinnamon Coffee Cake and the Nutty Caramel Logs!" (Susan M.)

"The Coffee Cake and Spice Cake are as good as any non-SCD recipe. The Herb Parmesan Bread has finally got me back to making sandwiches and ENJOYING them." (Deanna W.)

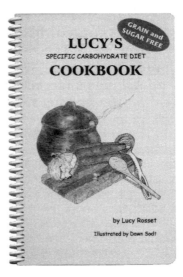

GRAIN and SUGAR FREE

LUCY'S
SPECIFIC CARBOHYDRATE DIET
COOKBOOK

by Lucy Rosset
Illustrated by Dawn Sodt

Other recommended cookbooks:

Recipes for the Specific Carbohydrate Diet by Raman Prasad
www.scdrecipe.com

Eat Well Feel Well by Kendall Conrad
www.eatwellfeelwellthebook.com

Grain-free Gourmet by Jodi Bager and Jenny Lass
www.grainfreegourmet.com

Healing Foods by Sandra Ramacher
www.ccccibs.com

The Juice Dilemma

During 1991, a leading commercial juice manufacturer had been found guilty of mislabeling their fruit juices. Their labels stated that there was no sugar, corn syrup, or sweetener added, but it was found that this labeling was deceptive. There have been many incidents like this in the past relating to fruit juice labeling. This is unfortunate because some companies are reliable, but it is beyond the scope of this book to check them all out. We have requested and received written assurance that Welch's 100% grape juice and Dole pineapple and pineapple-orange juices contain no added sugars. Additionally, Black River Juice Company (Canada) and Knudsen (U.S.A. and Canada) have confirmed their juices have no added sugars. These juices may be used in addition to apple cider (not apple juice) from a local cider mill (after you have talked to the owner) and juices that you squeeze yourself. We realize that there are many juice companies who are honest in their labeling and we suggest that, should you want to use any of them, you do your own detective work by calling and asking for a letter to back up statements on their labels, specifically, that no sweeteners have been added.

Dry Curd or Pressed Cottage Cheese

It has been advised in Chapter 9 that you should try to find a source of dry curd cottage cheese. This type of cheese is known by different names throughout the world. In some regions it is called "farmer's cheese" while in other areas, it is called "baker's cheese." No matter what it is called, it shares certain characteristics: (1) It is a white dry curd which has not had additional fluid added to it; (2) Since it has been separated from the lactose-rich whey and has been treated with a bacterial culture which eliminates residual lactose, its lactose content is very low. In some areas it is packed in plastic bags while in others places it is packed in containers containing about one cup. Sometimes it can be purchased in larger containers which can be divided into suitable serving sizes, and frozen to be taken out of the freezer as it is needed.

One of the Canadian producers of this product, Western Dairy (Western Creamery), distributes throughout parts of Canada. Western Dairy manufactures one of their products without the coagulating enzyme, rennin, which makes it suitable for the Muslim and Orthodox Jewish communities.

To help you obtain this product, local dairies and bakeries should be contacted to see if it can be purchased locally. If you are unsuccessful, the following information is offered to help you obtain this product which is used in recipes for cheese cake, Lois Lang's Luscious Bread, etc.

CANADA

Western Creamery, Inc.
2-91 Delta Park Blvd., Brampton, Ontario L6T 5E7
Toll free number: 1-800-265-3230
Website: www.WesternCreamery.com

Visit the website or call the toll-free number for more information on the products. People interested in purchasing dry curd products will be directed to the nearest retail location.

USA

Friendship Dairies
Product: FRIENDSHIP FARMER'S CHEESE
Telephone 1-516-719-4000 ask for customer service.
Email: myfriends@friendshipdairies.com
Or visit their website at www.friendshipdairies.com.

REFERENCES

Chapter 1: Past and Present

1. Haas, S.V. and M.P.Haas. 1951. *Management of Celiac Disease*. J.B. Lippincott Co., Philadelphia.
2. Dohan, F.C. 1966. Cereals and schizophrenia – data and hypotheses. Acta Psychiatry Scandinavia 42:125-152.
3. Dohan, F.C. 1978. Schizophrenia: Are some food-derived polypeptides pathogenic? In *The Biological Basis of Schizophrenia*. Eds. G. Hemmings and W.A. Hemmings. University Park Press, Baltimore.
4. Worthen, D. B. and J. R. Lorimer. 1979. *Enteral Hyperalimentation with Chemically Defined Elemental Diets: A Source Book*, 2nd ed. NorwichEaton Pharmaceuticals, Norwich, New York.
5. Russell, R.I. 1981. *Elemental Diets*. CRC Press, Florida.
6. Morin, C.L., M. Roulet, C.C. Roy, and A. Weber. 1980. Continuous elemental enteral alimentation in children with Crohn's disease and growth failure. Gastroenterology 79:1205-1210.
7. Sandberg, D.H., P.M. Tocci, and R.M. McKey. 1974. Decrease in sweat sodium chloride concentrations on limited diets. Pediatric Research 8:386.

Chapter 2: Scientific Evidence Relating to Diet

1. Haas, S.V. and M.P. Haas. 1951. *Management of Celiac Disease*. J. B. Lippincott Co., Philadelphia.
2. deDombal, F.T. 1968. Ulcerative colitis: definition, historical background, etiology, diagnosis, natural history and local complications. Postgraduate Medical journal 44:684-692.
3. Herter, C. 1908. *On Infantilism from Chronic Intestinal Infection*. MacMillan, New York.
4. Herter, C. 1910. Observations on intestinal infantilism. Transactions of the Association of American Physicians 25:528.
5. Gee, S. 1888. On the coeliac affliction. St. Bartholomew's Hospital Report 24:17.
6. Cozzetto, F.J. 1963. Intestinal lactase deficiency in a patient with cystic fibrosis. Report of a case with enzyme assay. Pediatrics 32:228-233.
7. Jones, R.H.T. 1964. Disaccharide intolerance and mucoviscidosis. Lancet 2:120-121.
8. Donaldson, R.M.,Jr. and J.D. Grybsoki. 1973. Carbohydrate intolerance. In *Gastrointestinal Disease*. Eds. M.H. Sleisenger and J.S. Fordtran. W.B. Saunders Co., Philadelphia.

9. Sandberg, D.H., P.M. Tocci, and R.M. McKey. 1974. Decrease in sweat sodium chloride concentrations on limited diets. Pediatric Research 8:386.

10. Struthers, J.E.,Jr., J.W.Singleton, and F. Kern,Jr. 1965. Intestinal lactase deficiency in ulcerative colitis and regional ileitis. Annals of Internal Medicine 63:221-228.

11. Wright, R., and S.C. Truelove. 1965. A controlled therapeutic trial of various diets in ulcerative colitis. British Medical journal 2:138-141.

12. Cady, A.B., J.B. Rhodes, A. Littman, and R.K. Crane. 1967. Significance of lactase deficit in ulcerative colitis. Journal of Laboratory and Clinical Medicine 70:279-286.

13. Kirschner, B.S., M.V. DeFavaro, and W. Jensen. 1981. Lactose malabsorption in children and adolescents with inflammatory bowel disease. Gastroenterology 81:829-832.

14. Truelove, S.C. 1961. Ulcerative colitis provoked by milk. British Medical journal 1:154-160.

15. McMichael, H.B., J. Webb, and A.M. Dawson. 1965. Lactase deficiency in adults: A cause of "functional" diarrhoea. Lancet 1:717-720.

16. Chalfin, D. and P.R. Holt. 1967. Lactase deficiency in ulcerative colitis, regional enteritis and viral hepatitis. American Journal of Digestive Diseases 12:81-87.

17. Gudmand-Hoyer, E. and S. Jarnum. 1970. Incidence and clinical significance of lactose malabsorption in ulcerative colitis and Crohn's disease. Gut 11:338-343.

18. Tandon, R., H. Mandell, H. M. Spiro, and W. R.,Thayer. 1971. Lactose intolerance in Jewish patients with ulcerative colitis. American journal of Digestive Diseases 16:845-848.

19. VonBrandes, J.W., and H. Lorenz-Meyer. 1981. Diet excluding refined sugar: a new perspective for the treatment of Crohn's disease? A randomized controlled study. Z. Gastroenterologie 19:1-12.

20. Alun Jones, A., E. Workman, A.H. Freeman, R.J. Dickinson, A.J. Wilson, and J.O. Hunter. 1985. Crohn's disease: Maintenance of remission by diet. Lancet 11: 177-180.

21. Morin, C.L., M. Roulet, C.C. Roy, and A. Weber. 1980. Continuous elemental enteral alimentation in children with Crohn's disease and growth failure. Gastroenterology 79:1205-1210.

22. VanEys, J. 1977. Nutritional therapy in children with cancer. Cancer Research 37:2457-2461.

23. Poley, J.R. 1984. Ultrastructural topography of small bowel mucosa in chronic diarrhea in infants and children: Investigations with the scanning electron microscope. In *Chronic Diarrhea in Children*. Ed. E. Lebenthal. Nestle, Vevey/Raven Press, New York.

24. Salyers, A.A. 1979. Energy sources of major intestinal fermentative anaerobes. American Journal of Clinical Nutrition 32:158-163.

25. McCarrison, R. 1922. Faulty food in relation to gastrointestinal disorders. JAMA 78:1-8.

26. Heaton, K.W. 1990. Dietary factors in the aetiology of inflammatory bowel disease. In *Inflammatory Bowel Diseases*. Eds. R.N. Allan, M.R.B Keighley, J. Alexander-Williams, and C.E Hawkins. Churchill Livingstone, New York.

Chapter 3: Intestinal Microbes: The Unseen World

1. Bengson, M.H. 1979. Effects of bioisolation on the intestinal microflora. American Journal of Clinical Nutrition 23:1525-1532.
2. Ropeloff, N. 1930. *Man Versus Microbes*. Garden City Publishing Co., Inc., Garden City, New York.
3. Haenel, H. 1970. Human normal and abnormal gastrointestinal flora. American Journal of Clinical Nutrition 23:1433-1439.
4. Shahani, K.M. and A.D. Ayebo. 1980. Role of dietary lactobacilli in gastrointestinal microecology. American journal of Clinical Nutrition 33:2448-2457.
5. Simon, G.L. and S.L. Gorbach. 1981. Intestinal flora in health and disease. In *Physiology of the Gastrointestinal Tract*, Vol.2. Ed. L.R. Johnson. Raven Press, New York.
6. Feibusch, J.M. and P.R. Holt. 1982. Impaired absorptive capacity for carbohydrate in the aging human. Digestive Diseases and Sciences 27:1095-1100.
7. Gracey, M.S. 1981. Nutrition, bacteria and the gut. British Medical Bulletin 37:71-75.
8. McEvoy, A., J. Dutton, and O.F.W.James. 1983. Bacterial contamination of the small intestine is an important cause of occult malabsorption in the elderly. British Medical journal 287:789-793.
9. Dubos, R. 1962. *The Unseen World*. The Rockefeller Institute Press, New York.
10. Pope, C.II. 1983. Involvement of the esophagus by infections, systemic illnesses and physical agents. In *Gastrointestinal Disease*. Eds. M.H. Sleisenger and J.S. Fordtran. W. B. Saunders Co., Philadelphia.
11. Rolfe, R.D. and S.M. Finegold. 1980. Inhibitory interactions between normal fecal flora and Clostridium difficile. American journal of Clinical Nutrition 33:2539.
12. Donaldson, R.M. 1964. Normal bacterial populations of the intestine and their relation to intestinal function. The New England Journal of Medicine 270:938-945.
13. King, C.E. and P.E. Toskes. 1979. Small intestine bacterial overgrowth. Gastroenterology 76:1035-1055.
14. Haas, S.V. and M.P. Haas. 1951. *Management of Celiac Disease*. J.B. Lippincott Co., Philadelphia.
15. Flexner, S. and J.E. Sweet. 1906. The pathogenesis of experimental colitis and the relation of colitis in animals and man. journal of Experimental Medicine 8:514-535.
16. Morgan, H.D. 1907. Upon the bacteriology of the summer diarrhea of infants. British Medical journal 2:16-19.

17. Bassler, A. 1922. Treatment of cases of ulcerative colitis. Medical Record 101:227-229.
18. Bargen, J.A. 1924. Experimental studies on etiology of chronic ulcerative colitis.)AMA 83:332-336.
19. Crohn, B.B., L. Ginzburg, and G.D. Oppenheimer. 1932. Regional ileitis. JAMA 99:1323-1329.
20. Menon, T.B. 1930. The pathology of chronic colitis in the tropics. Indian Journal of Medical Research 18:137-141.
21. Bargen, J.A., M.C. Copeland, L.A. Buie. 1931. The relation of dysentery bacilli to chronic ulcerative colitis. Practitioner 127:235-247.
22. Hurst, A.F. 1931. Ulcerative colitis. Proceedings of the Royal Society of Medicine 24:785-803.
23. Felsen, J. and W. Wolarsky. 1953. Acute and chronic bacillary dysentery and chronic ulcerative colitis. JAMA 153:1069-1072.
24. Takeuchi, A., S.B. Formal, and H. Sprinz. 1968. Acute colitis in Rhesus monkey following peroral infection with Shigella flexneri. American Journal of Pathology 52:503-529.
25. Staley, T.E., L.D. Corley, and E.W. Jones. 1970. Early pathogenesis of colitis in neonatal pigs monocontaminated with Escherichia coli. Fine structural changes in the colonic epithelium. American Journal of Digestive Diseases 15:923-935.
26. DuPont, H.I., S.B. Formal, R.B. Hornick, M.J. Snyder, J.P. Libonati, D.G. Sheahan, E.H. LaBrec, and J.P. Kalas. 1971. Pathogenesis of Escherichia coli diarrhea. The New England Journal of Medicine 285:1-9.
27. Metchnikoff, E. 1908. *The Prolongation of Life*. G.P. Putnam's Sons, New York.
28. Robins-Browne, R.M. and M.M. Levine. 1981. The fate of ingested lactobacilli in the proximal small intestine. American Journal of Clinical Nutrition 34:514-519.
29. Kolars, J.C. M.D. Levitt, M.M. Aouji, and D.A. Savaino. 1984. Yogurt - an autodigesting source of lactose. New England Journal of Medicine 310:1-3.
30. McCarrison, R. 1922. Faulty food in relation to gastrointestinal disorders. JAMA 78:1-8.
31. Necheles, H. and C. Beck. 1965. Lactobacillus and intestinal flora. Applied Therapeutics 7:463-465.
32. Sandine, W.E., K.S. Muralidhara, P.R. Elliker, and D.C. England. 1972. Lactic acid bacteria in food and health. Journal of Milk and Food Technology 35:691-702.
33. Johnson, W.C. 1974. Oral elemental diet. Archives of Surgery 108:32-34.
34. George, W.L., R.D. Rolfe, V.L. Sutter, and S.M. Finegold. 1979. Diarrhea and colitis associated with antimicrobial therapy in man and animals. American Journal of Clinical Nutrition 32:251-257.

35. Willoughby, J.M.T. 1982. The alimentary system. In *Iatrogenic Diseases*, 2nd ed. Eds. P.P. D'Arcy and J.P. Griffin. Oxford University Press, New York.
36. Ziv, G.M., M.J. Paape, and A.M. Dulin. 1983. Influence of antibiotics and intramammary antibiotic products on phagocytosis of Staphylococcus aureaus by bovine leukocytes. American Journal of Veterinary Research 44:385-388.
37. Low-Beer, T.S. and A.E. Reed. 1971. Progress report. Diarrhoea: Mechanisms and treatment. Gut 12:1021-1036.
38. Keusch, G.T., and D.H. Present. 1976. Summary of a workshop on clindamycin colitis. Journal of infectious Diseases 133:578-587.
39. Toffler, R.B., E.G. Pingoud, and M.I. Burrell. 1978. Acute colitis related to penicillin and penicillin derivatives. Lancet 2:707-709.
40. Sakurai, Y., H. Tsuchiya, F. Ikegami, T. Funatomi, S. Takasu, and T. Uchikoshi. 1979. Acute right-sided hemorrhagic colitis associated with oral administration of ampicillin. Digestive Diseases and Sciences 24:910-915.
41. Boriello, S.P., R.H. Jones, and I. Phillips. 1980. Rifampicin-associated pseudomembranous colitis. British Medical journal 281:1180-1181.
42. Fournier, G., J. Orgiazzi, B. Lenoir, and M. Dechavannne. Pseudomembranous colitis probably due to rifampicin. Lancet 1:101.
43. Friedman, R.J., I.E. Mayer, J.T. Galambos, and T. Hersh. 1980. Oxacillin-induced pseudomembranous colitis. American Journal of Gastroenterology 72:445-447.
44. Saginur, R., C.R. Hawley, and J.G. Bartlett. 1980. Colitis-associated metronidazole therapy. Journal of infectious Disease 141:772-774.
45. Thomson, G., A.H. Clark, K. Hare, and W.G.S. Spilg. 1981. Pseudomembranous colitis after treatment with metronidazole. British Medical journal 282:864-865.
46. Weidema, W.F., M.F. Von Meyenfeidt, P.B. Soeters, R.I.C. Wesdorp, and J.M. Greep. 1980. Pseudomembranous colitis after whole gut irrigation with neomycin and erythromycin base. British journal of Surgery 67:895-896.
47. Coleman, D.L. P.H. Juergensen, M.H. Brand, and F.O. Finkelstein. 1981. Antibiotic-associated diarrhoea during administration of intraperitoneal cephalothin. Lancet 1:1004.
48. Lishman, A.H., I.J. Al-Jumaili, and C.O.Record. 1981. Spectrum of antibiotic-associated diarrhoea. Gut 22:34-37.
49. Taylor, A.G. 1976. Toxins and the genesis of specific lesions: Enterotoxin and exfoliatin. In *Mechanisms in Bacterial Toxicology*. Ed. A.W. Bernheimer. John Wiley and Sons, New York.
50. Arbuthnott, J.P. and C.J. Smith. 1979. Bacterial adhesion in host/pathogen interactions in animals. In *Adhesion of Microorganisms to Surfaces*. Eds. D.C. Ellwood and J. Melling. Academic Press, London.

51. Salyers, A.A. 1979. Energy sources of major intestinal fermentative anaerobes. American Journal of Clinical Nutrition 32:158-163.

52. Moore, W.E.C. and L.V. Holdeman. 1975. Discussion of current bacteriological investigations of the relationships between intestinal flora, diet, and colon cancer. Cancer Research 35:3418-3420.

Chapter 4: Breaking the Vicious Cycle

1. Stephen, A.M. 1985. Effect of food on the intestinal microflora. *In Food and the Gut.* Eds. J.O. Hunter and V.A. Jones. Bailliere Tindall, London.

2. Weijers, H.A. and J.H. vandeKamer. 1965. Treatment of malabsorption of carbohydrates. Modern Treatment 2:378-390.

3. Oh, M.S., K.R. Phelps, M.Traube, J.L. Barbosa-Salvidar, C. Boxhill, and H.J. Carroll. 1979. D-Lactic acidosis in a man with the short-bowel syndrome. New England Journal of Medicine 301:249-252.

4. Stolberg, L., R. Rolfe, N. Gitlin, J. Merritt, L. Mann, J. Linder, and S. Finegold. 1982. D-Lactic acidosis due to abnormal gut flora. New England Journal of Medicine 306:1344-1348.

5. Traube, M., J. Bock, and J.L. Boyer. 1982. D-Lactic acidosis after jejunoileal bypass. New England Journal of Medicine 307:1027.

6. Lifshitz, F. 1982. Necrotizing enterocolitis and feedings. In *Pediatric Nutrition.* Ed. F. Lifshitz. Marcel Dekker, Inc., New York.

7. Jonas, A., P.R. Flanagan, and G.C. Forstner. 1977. Pathogenesis of mucosal injury in the blind loop syndrome. journal of Clinical Investigation 60:1321-1330.

8. Lee, P.C. 1984. Transient carbohydrate malabsorption and intolerance in diarrheal diseases of infancy. In *Chronic Diarrhea in Children.* Ed. E. Lebenthal. Nestle, Vevey/Raven Press, New York.

9. Johnson, W.C. 1974. Oral elemental diet. Archives of Surgery 108:32-34.

10. Jarnum, S. 1976. Chemically defined diets in medicine. Nutrition and Metabolism 20 (Supplement 1):19-26.

11. Diez-Gonzalez, F., T.R. Callaway, M.G. Kizoulis, and J.B. Russell. 1998. Grain feeding and dissemination of acid-resistant Escherichia coli from cattle. Science 281:1666-1668.

12. Pai, C.H., R. Gordon, H.V. Sims, et al. 1984. Sporadic cases of hemorrhagic colitis associated with Escherichia coli 0157:H7. Annals of Internal Medicine 101:738-742.

13. Riley, L.W., R.S. Remis, S.D. Helgerson, et al. 1983. Hemorrhagic colitis associated with a rare Escherichia coli serotype. New England Journal of Medicine 308:681-685.

14. Burke, D.A. and A.T.R. Axon. 1987. Ulcerative colitis and Escherichia coli with adhesive properties. Journal of Clinical Pathology 40:782786.

Chapter 5: Carbohydrate Digestion

1. Go, V.L.W. and W.H.J. Summerskill. 1971. Digestion, maldigestion, and the gastrointestinal hormones. American Journal of Clinical Nutrition. 24:160-167.
2. Gee, S. 1888. On the coeliac affliction. St. Bartholomew Hospital Report 24:17.
3. Moog, F. 1981. The lining of the small intestine. Scientific American 245:154-176.
4. Poley, J. R. 1984. Ultrastructural topography of small bowel mucosa in chronic diarrhea in infants and children: Investigations with the scanning electron microscope. In *Chronic Diarrhea in Children*. Ed. E. Lebenthal. Nestle, Vevey/Raven Press, New York.
5. Plotkin, G.R. and K.J. Isselbacher. 1964. Secondary disaccharidase deficiency in adult celiac disease (non tropical sprue) and other malabsorption states. New England journal of Medicine. 271:1033-1037.
6. Burke, V., K.R. Kerry, and C.M. Anderson. 1965. The relationship of dietary lactose to refractory diarrhea in infancy. Australian Paediatric journal 1:147-160.
7. Kojecky, Z. and Z. Matlocha. 1965. Quantitative differences of intestinal disaccharidase activity following the resection of stomach. Gastroenterologia (Basel) 104:343-351.
8. McMichael, H.B., J. Webb, and A.M. Dawson. 1965. Lactase deficiency in adults: a cause of functional diarrhoea. Lancet 1:717:720.
9. Weser, E. and M.H. Sleisenger. 1965. Lactosuria and lactase deficiency in adult celiac disease. Gastroenterology 48:571-578.
10. Weser, E., W. Rubin, L. Ross, and M.H. Sleisenger. 1965. Lactase deficiency in patients with the "irritable-colon syndrome." New England Journal of Medicine 273:1070-1075.
11. Welsh, J.D., O.M. Zschiesche, J. Anderson, and A. Walker. 1969. Intestinal disaccharidase activity in celiac sprue (gluten-sensitive enteropathy). Archives of Internal Medicine 123:33-38.
12. Prinsloo, J.G., W. Wittmann, H. Kruger, E. Freier. 1971. Lactose absorption and mucosal disaccharidases in convalescent pellagra and kwashiorkor children. Archives of Diseases of Childhood 46:474-478.
13. King, E. and P.P. Toskes. 1979. Small intestine bacterial overgrowth. Gastroenterology 76:1035-1055.
14. Gray, G. 1982. Intestinal disaccharidase deficiencies and glucose-galactose malabsorption. In *The Metabolic Basis of Inherited Disease*. Eds. J.B.Stanbury, J.B.Wyngaarden, D.S.Fredrickson, J.S.Goldstein, and M.S.Brown. 5th ed. McGraw-Hill Book Co., New York.

15. Campos, J.V,M., U.F. Neto, F.R.S. Patricio, J. Wehba, A.A. Carvalho, and M. Shiner. 1979. Jejunal mucosa in marasmic children. Clinical, pathological, and fine structural evaluation of the effect of protein-energy malnutrition and environmental contamination. American Journal of Clinical Nutrition. 32:1575-1591.

16. Brunser, O. and M. Araya. 1984. Damage and repair of small intestinal mucosa in acute and chronic diarrhea. In *Chronic Diarrhea in Children*. Ed. E. Lebenthal. Nestle Vevey/Raven Press, New York.

17. Dvorak, A.M., A.B. Connell, and G. R. Dickersin. 1979. Crohn's disease: A scanning electron microscopic study. Human Pathology 10:165-177.

18. Lee, P.C. 2984. Transient carbohydrate malabsorption and intolerance in diarrhea disease of infancy. In *Chronic Diarrhea of Children*. Ed. E. Lebenthal. Nestle, Vevey/Raven Press, New York.

19. Pope, C.E. 11. 1983. Involvement of the esophagus by infections, systemic illnesses and physical agents. In *Gastrointestinal Disease*. Eds. M.H. Sleisenger and J.S. Fordtran. W. B. Saunders Co., Philadelphia.

20. Anderson, I.H., A.S. Levine, and M.D. Levitt. 1981. Incomplete absorption of the carbohydrate in all-purpose wheat flour. New England Journal of Medicine 304:891-892.

21. Feibusch, J.M. and P.R. Holt. 1982. Impaired absorptive capacity for carbohydrate in the aging human. Digestive diseases and Sciences 27:1095-1100.

22. Rackis, J.J. 1975. Oligosaccharides of food legumes: Alpha-galactosidase activity and the flatus problem. In *Physiological Effects of Food Carbohydrates*. Eds. A. Jeanes and J. Hodge. American Chemical Society, Washington, D.C.

23. Fisher, S.E., G. Leone, R.H. Kelly. 1981. Chronic protracted diarrhea: Intolerance to dietary glucose polymers. Pediatrics 67:271-273.

24. Lebenthal, E., L. Heitlinger, P.C. Lee, K.S. Nord, C. Holdge, S.P. Brooks, and D. George. 1983. Corn syrup sugars: In vitro and in vivo digestibility and clinical tolerance in acute diarrhea of infancy. Journal of Pediatrics 103:29-34.

25. Juliano, B.O. 1972. Physicochemical properties of starch and protein in relation to grain quality and nutritional value of rice. Internation Rice Research Institute (Los Banos) Annual Report.

26. Weiner, M. and J. VanEys. 1983. In *Nicotinic Acid*. Marcel Dekker, Inc. New York.

27. Cooke, W.T. and G.K.T. Holmes. 1984. *Coeliac Disease*. Churchill Livingstone, New York.

28. Gunja-Smith, Z., J.J. Marshall, C. Mercier, E.E. Smith, and W.J. Whelan. 1970. A revision of the Meyer-Bernfield model of glycogen and amylopectin. FEBS Letters 12:101-104.

29. Davidson, G.P. and R.R.W. Townley. 1977. Structural and functional abnormalities of the small intestine due to nutritional folic acid deficiency in infancy. journal of Paediatrics 90:590-595.

Chapter 6: The Celiac Story

1. Crichton, M. 1968. *A Case of Need*. Penguin Books, New York, p. 84.
2. Aretaeus the Cappadocian. 1856. On the *Cause and Symptoms of Chronic Disease*. The Sydenham Society, London.
3. Gull, W. 1853, Fatty Stools from Disease of the Mesenteric Glands. Guy's Hospital Report 1:369.
4. Gee, S. 1888. On the Coeliac Affection. St. Bartholomew's Hospital Report 24:17.
5. Herter, C. 1908. *On Infantilism from Chronic Intestinal Infection*. MacMillan, New York.
6. Newland, J. 1921. Prolonged intolerance to carbohydrates. Transactions of American Pediatric Society. 44:11.
7. Golden Jubiliee World Tribute to Dr. Sidney V. Haas. 1949. *The Story of Dr. Sidney V. Haas*. New York Academy of Medicine, New York.
8. Haas, S.V. and M.P. Haas. 1951 *Management of Celiac Disease*. J. B. Lippincott Company, Philadelphia. p.x
9. Editorial, April 5, 1949. *New York Times*. p. 28, col. 2
10. Physicians Honor Pediatric Pioneer. April 6, 1949. *New York Times*. p. 34, col. 2
11. Haas, S.V. and M.P. Haas. 1951. *Management of Celiac Disease*. J. B. Lippincott Company, Philadelphia.
12. Anderson, C.M., J.M. French, H.H. Sammons, A.C, Frazer, J.W. Gerrard, and J.M. Smellie. 1952. Coeliac disease: Gastrointestinal studies and the effect of dietary wheat flour. Lancet 1: 836-842
13. Matthews, D.M. 1975. Intestinal absorption of peptides. Physiological Review 55:537-608.
14. Moog, F. 1981. The lining of the small intestine. Scientific American 245:154-176.
15. Cluysenaer,.O.J.J. and J.H.M.vanTongeren. 1977. *Malabsorption in Coeliac Sprue*. Martinus Nijhoff Medical Division, Hague.
16. Phelan, J.J., F.M.Stevens, W.F. Cleere, B. McNicholl, C.F. McCarthy, and P.F. Fottrell. 1978. The detoxification of gliadin by the enzymic cleavage of a side-chain substituent. In *Perspectives in Coeliac Disease*. Eds. B. McNicholl, C.F. McCarthy and P.F. Fottrell. University Park Press, Baltimore.
17. Stevens, F.M., J.J. Phelan, B. McNicholl, F.R. Comerford, P.F. Fottrell, and C.F. McCarthy. 1978. Clinical demonstration of the reduction of gliadin toxicity by enzymic cleavage of side-chain substituent. In *Perspectives in Coeliac Disease*. Eds. B. McNicholl, C.F. McCarthy, and P.F. Fottrell. University Park Press, Baltimore.
18. Anderson, I.H., A.S. Levine, and M.D. Levitt. 1981. Incomplete absorption of the carbohydrate in all purpose wheat flour. New England Journal of Medicine 304:891-892.
19. Cooke, W.T. and G.K.T. Holmes. 1984. *Coeliac Disease*. Churchill Livingstone, New York.

20. Congdon, P., M.K. Mason, S. Smith, A. Crollick, A. Steel, and J. Littlewood. 1981 Small bowel mucosa in asymptomatic children with celiac disease. American Journal of Disease in Children 135:118-122.

21. Rubin, C.E., L.L. Brandborg, A.L. Flick, P. Phelps, C. Parmentier, and S. van Niel. 1962. Studies in celiac sprue. III. The effect of repeated wheat instillation into the proximal ileum of patients on a gluten-free diet. Gastroenterology 43:621-641.

22. Bleumink, E., 1974. Allergens and toxic protein in food. In *Coeliac Disease*. Eds. W.T.J.M. Hekkens and A.S. Peña. Stenfert Kroese. Leiden.

23. Weiser, M.M. 1976. An alternative mechanism for gluten toxicity in coeliac disease. Lancet 1:567-569.

24. Baker, P.G. and A.E. Read. 1976. Oats and barley toxicity in celiac patients. Postgraduate Medical Journal 52:264-268.

25. Strunk, R.C., J.L. Pinnas, T.J. John, R.C. Hansen, and J.L. Blazovich. 1978. Rice hypersensitivity associated with serum complement depression. Clinical Allergy 8:51-58.

26. Vitoria, J.C., C. Camarero, A. Sojo, A. Ruiz, and J. Rodriguez-Soriano. 1982. Enteropathy related to fish, rice, and chicken. Archives of Disease in Childhood 57:44-48.

27. Kagnoff, M.F. 1995. Celiac disease. In *Textbook of Gastroenterology*. Vol. 2. Eds. T. Yamada et al. J.B. Lippincott Company, Philadelphia. p., 1644.

28. Creamer, B. 1966. Coeliac thoughts. Gut 7:569-571.

29. Poley, J.R. 1984. Ultrastructural topography of small bowel mucosa in chronic diarrhea in infants and children: Investigations with the scanning electron microscope. In *Chronic Diarrhea in Children*. Ed. E. Lebenthal. Nestle, Vevey/Raven Press, New York.

30. King, C.E. and P.P. Toskes. 1979. Small intestine bacterial overgrowth. Gastroenterology 76:1035-1055.

31. Araya, M. and J.A. Walker-Smith. 1975. Specificity of ultrastructural changes of small intestinal epithelium in early childhood. Archives of Disease in Childhood 50:844-855.

32. Brunser, O. and M. Araya. 1984. Damage and repair of small intestinal mucosa in acute and chronic diarrhea. In Chronic Diarrhea in Children. Ed. E. Lebenthal. Nestle Vevey/Raven Press, New York.

33. Holmes, G.K.T., P.L. Stokes, T.M. Sorahan, P. Prior, J.A.H. Waterhouse, and W.T. Cooke. 1976. Coeliac disease, gluten free diet, and malignancy. Gut 17:612-619.

34. Lifshitz, F. and G. Holman. 1966. Familial celiac disease with intestinal disaccharidase deficiencies. American journal of Digestive Diseases 11:377-387.

35. Berg, N.O., A. Dahlqvist, T. Lindberg, and A. Norden. 1970. Intestinal dipeptidases and disaccharidases in celiac disease in adults. Gastroenterology 59:575-582.

36. Plotkin, G.R. and K.J. Isselbacher. 1964. Secondary disaccharidase deficiency in adult celiac disease (non tropical sprue) and other malabsorption states. New England Journal of Medicine 271:1033-1037.
37. Townley, R.R.W., K.T. Khaw, and H. Schwachman. 1965. Quantitative assay of disaccharidase activities of small intestinal mucosal biopsy specimens in infancy and childhood. Pediatrics 36:911-921.
38. Arthur, A.B. 1966. Intestinal disaccharidase deficiency in children with celiac disease. Archives of Diseases in Children 41:519-524.
39. Littman, A. and J.B. Hammond. 1965. Diarrhoea in adults caused by deficiency in intestinal disaccharidases. Gastroenterology 48:237-249.
40. Personal correspondence (unpublished). Nov. 6, 1996. From Jennifer Stenberg to Elaine Gottschall. Writer's address; R. R. 1., Holstein, Ont., Canada. NOG 2A0.

Chapter 7: The Brain Connection

1. Cooke, WT. and WT. Smith. 1966. Neurological disorders associated with adult coeliac disease. Brain 89:683-722.
2. Gracey, M.S. 1981. Nutrition, bacteria, and the gut. British Medical Bulletin 37:71-75.
3. McEvoy, A.J., J. Dutton, and O.F. W James. 1983. Bacterial contamination of the small intestine is an important cause of occult malabsorption in the elderly. British Medical journal 287:789-793.
4. Dakshinamurti, K. 1982. Neurobiology of pyrodoxine. In *Advances in Nutritional Research* Vol. 4. Ed. H. Draper. Plenum Press, New York.
5. Levenson, A.J. 1983. Organic brain syndromes, other nonfunctional psychiatric disorders, and pseudodementia. In *Fundamentals of Geriatric Medicine*. Eds. R.D.T. Cape, R.M. Coe, and 1. Rossman. Raven Press, New York.
6. Baruk, H. 1978. Psychoses from digestive origins. In *The Biological Basis of Schizophrenia*. Eds. G. and W H. Hemmings. University Park Press, Baltimore.
7. Buscaino, G.A. 1978. The amino-hepato-entero-toxic theory of schizophrenia: an historical review. In *The Biological Basis of Schizophrenia*. Eds. G. and W.H. Hemmings. University Park Press, Baltimore.
8. Dohan, EC. 1966. Cereals and schizophrenia-data and hypotheses. Acta Psychiatry Scandinavia 42:125-152.
9. Hunter, J.0.1991. Food allergy-or enterometabolic disorder? The Lancet 338:495-496.
10. Truss, C. Orian. 1983. *The Missing Diagnosis*, R O. Box 26508, Birmingham, Alabama 35226.
11. Stephen, A.M. 1985. Effect of food on the intestinal microflora. In *Food and the Gut*. Eds. J.0. Hunter and V .A. Jones. Bailhere Tindall, London.

12. Man S. Oh, K.R. Phelps, M. Traube, J.L. Barbosa-Salvidar, C. Boxhill, and H.J. Carroll. 1979. D-lactic acidosis in a man with the short-bowel syndrome. The New England Journal of Medicine 301:249-252.
13. Stolberg, L., R. Rolfe, N. Gitlin, J. Merritt, L. Mann, Jr., J. Linder, and S. Finegold. 1982. D-lactic acidosis due to abnormal flora. The New England journal of medicine 306:13441348.
14. Perlmutter, D.H., J.T. Boyle, J.M. Campos, J.M. Egler, and J.B. Watkins, 1983. D-lactic acidosis in children: an unusual metabolic complication of small bowel resection. The journal of Pediatrics 102:234-238.
15. Haan, E., G. Brown, A. Bankier, D. Mitchell, S. Hunt, J. Blakey, and G. Barnes. 1985. Severe illness caused by the products of bacterial metabolism in a child with a short gut. European journal of Pediatrics 144:63-65.
16. Traube, M., J. Bock, and J.L. Boyer. 1982. D-lactic acidosis after jenunoileal bypass. The New England journal of Medicine 307:1027.
17. Mayne, A.J., D.J. Handy, M.A. Preece, R.H. George, and I.W. Booth. 1990. Dietary management of D-lactic acidosis in short bowel syndrome. Archives of Diseases of Childhood 65:229-231.
18. Thurn, J.R., G.L. Pierpont, C.W Ludvigsen, and J.H. Eckfeldt. 1985. D-lactate encephalopathy. The American journal of medicine 79:717721.

Chapter 8: The Autism Connection

1. Ashwood, P., S.H. Murch, A. Anthony., A. A. Pellicer, F. Torrente, M.A. Thomson, J.A. Walker-Smith, and A.J. Wakefield. 2003. Intestinal lymphocyte populations in children with regressive autism: Evidence for extensive mucosal immunopathology. Journal of Clinical Immunology 23(6):504-517.
2. Buie, T., H. Winter and R. Kushak. 2002. Preliminary findings in gastrointestinal investigation of autistic patients.
3. J.O. Hunter. 1991. Food allergy or enterometabolic disorder. Lancet 338: 495-496.
4. Coleman, M. and J.P. Blass. 1985. Autism and lactic acidosis. Journal of Autism and Developmental Disorders. 15:1-8.Four patients are described who have two coexistent syndromes: the behavioral syndrome of autism and the biochemical syndrome of lactic acidosis. One of the four patients also had hyperuricemia and hyperuricosuria. These patients raise the possibility that one subgroup of the autism syndrome may be associated with inborn errors of carbohydrate metabolism.
5. Man S. Oh, K.R. Phelps, M. Traube, J.L. Barbosa-Salvidar, C. Boxhill, and H.J. Carroll. 1979. D-lactic acidosis in a man with the short-bowel syndrome. The New England Journal of Medicine 301:249-252.
6. Stolberg, L., R. Rolfe, N. Gitlin, J. Merritt, L. Mann, Jr., J. Linder, and S. Finegold. 1982. D-lactic acidosis due to abnormal flora. The New England Journal of Medicine 306:1344-1348.

7. Perlmutter, D.H., J.T. Boyle, J.M. Campos, J.M Egler, and J.B. Watkins, 1983. D-lactic acidosis in children: an unusual metabolic complication of small bowel resection. The Journal of Pediatrics 102:234-238.
8. Haan, E., G. Brown, A. Bankier, D. Mitchell, S. Hunt, J. Blakey, and G. Barnes. 1985. Severe illness caused by the products of bacterial metabolism in a child with a short gut. European Journal of Pediatrics 144:63-65.
9. Traube, M., J. Bock, and J.L. Boyer. 1982. D-lactic acidosis after jenunoileal bypass. The New England Journal of Medicine 307:1027.
10. Mayne, A.J., D.J. Handy, M.A. Preece, R.H. George, and I.W. Booth. 1990. Dietary management of D-lactic acidosis in short bowel syndrome. Archives of Diseases of Childhood 65:229-231.
11. Thurn, J.R., G.L. Pierpont, C.W. Ludvigsen, and J.H. Eckfeldt. 1985. D-lactate encephalopathy. The American Journal of Medicine 79:717-721.
12. Melmud, R., C. K. Schneider, R. A. Fabes, et al. 2000.Metabolic markers and gastrointestinal symptoms in children with autism and related disorders. Journal of Pediatric Gastroenterology and Nutrition. 31:A116.
13. Wakefield, A.J., S. H. Murch, A. Anthony, J. Linnell, D. M. Casson, M. Malik, M. Berclowitz, A.P. Dhillon, M. A. Thomson, P. Harvey, A. Valentine, S.E. Davies, and J. A. Walker-Smith. 1998. Ileal-lymphoid-nodular hyperplasia, non-specific colitis, and pervasive developmental disorder in children. Lancet 351: 637-41.
14. Wakefield, A.J., A. Anthony, S.H. Murch, M. Thomson, , S.M. Montgomer, S. Davies, J. J. O'Leary, m. Berelowitz, and J.A. Walker-Smith. 2000. Enterocolitis in children with developmental disorders. American Journal of Gastroenterology 95:2285-2295.
15. Hovarth, K., J.C. Papadimitriou, A. Rabsztyn, C. Drachenberg, and J. T. Tildon. 1999. Gastrointestinal abnormalities in children with autistic disorder. Journal of Pediatrics 135: 559-63.
16. Harvard Autism Project. 2002. Initial Autism Research Findings at Harvard Massachusetts General Hospital.
17. Wakefield, A. J. 2002. The gut-brain axis in childhood developmental disorders. In Journal of Pediatric Gastroenterology and Nutrition. Lippincott Williams & Wilkins, Inc., Philadelphia.
18. Butterworth, R. F. 2000. Complications of cirrhosis III hepatic Encephalopathy. Journal of Hepatology 32:171-180.
19. Bolte, E. R. 1998. Autism and Clostridium tetani. Medical Hypothesis 55:133-44.
20. Jyonouchi, H, S. Sun, and N. Itokazu. 2002. Innate immunity associated with inflammatory responses and cytokine production against common dietary proteins in patients with autism spectrum disorder. Neuropsychobiology 46:76-84.

21. Ulevitch, R.J. and P.S. Tobias. 1999. Recognition of gram-negative bacteria and endotoxin by the innate immune system. Current Opinions Immunology. 11:19-22. Until about 10 years ago the exact mechanisms controlling cellular responses to the endotoxin – or lipopolysaccharide (LPS) – of Gram-negative bacteria were unknown. Now a considerable body of evidence supports a model where LPS or LPS-containing particles (including intact bacteria) form complexes with a serum protein known as LPS-binding protein; the LPS in the complex is subsequently transferred to another protein which binds LPS, CD14. The latter is found on the plasma membrane of most cell types of the myeloid lineage as well as in the serum in its soluble form. LPS binding of these two forms of CD 14 results in the activation of cell types of myeloid and nonmyeloid lineages respectively.
22. Medzhitov, R. and C. Janeway. 2000. Innate immunity. The New England Journal of Medicine 343:338-344.

Chapter 9: Introducing the Diet

1. Haas, S.V. and M.P. Haas. 1951. *Management of Celiac Disease*. J.13. Lippincott Co., Philadelphia.
2. Kraybill, H.F. 1977. Nonoccupational environmental cancer. In *Advances in Modern Toxicology*. Vol. 3. John Wiley & Sons, New York.
3. Delmont, J. 1983. Milk consumption and rejection throughout the world. In *Milk Intolerance and Rejection*. Ed. J. Delmont. Karger, Basel.
4. Van Soest, P.J. 1981. Some factors influencing the ecology of gut fermentation in man. In *Banbury Report 7 – Gastrointestinal Cancer: Endogenous Factors*. Eds. W.R. Bruce, P. Correa, M. Lipkin, S.R.Tannenbaum, and T.D. Wilkins. Cold Spring Harbor Laboratory.
5. Connon, J.J. and K.N. Jeejeebhoy. 1985. General approach to acute and chronic diarrhea. In *Gastrointestinal Diseases*. Ed. K.N. Jeejeebhoy. Medical Examination Publishing Co., Inc., New Hyde Park, New York.

Gourmet Section

1. Fisher, S. E., G. Leone, R. H. Kelly. 1981. Chronic protracted diarrhea: Intolerance to dietary glucose polymers. Pediatrics 67:271-273.

INDEX

Not all food items have been listed in the index. For a complete listing of permitted foods, see Chapter 10, The Specific Carbohydrate Diet. References with Roman numerals, i-iv, are found in the Foreword.

Sucrase 25
Sucrose 3, 6, 7, 8, 22, 24, 25, 27, 28,
  57, 71, 76, 77, 181
Sugars 5, 6, 7, 8, 21, 24, 25, 26, 27,
  42, 47, 55, 57, 62, 63, 64, 65, 67,
  70, 71, 172, 180, 184
  (see Chapter 1, 10)
Sulfa drugs 1, 16
Sulfites 73
Sweat test for CF
  sodium chloride in perspiration 2
Sweeteners, artificial
  aspartame, (Nutri-Sweet, etc.) 75
  saccharin 62, 72, 74, 76, 78
  sorbitol 62
  xylitol 62
Synthetic diet (see Elemental diet)
T
Thrush, oral 26
Tofu 64
Toxicity, intestinal iii, 14, 15, 24, 33,
  38, 39, 46, 47
Toxins, microbial (yeast and
  bacterial)
  (see Toxicity)
Triticale 67, 72
Truss, Dr. C.O. 47

U
Ulcerative colitis 1, 5, 6, 7, 14, 19, 25,
  26, 41, 46, 48, 56, 70, 161, 163
V
Vagus nerve 57
Van Eys, Dr. J. 8
Vegetables 3, 27, 28, 29, 30, 36, 60,
  61, 63, 64, 69, 71, 72, 74, 167
Vegetarian diet 64
Vitamin A 65, 159
Vitamin B12 13, 24, 64, 65
Vitamin B-Complex 65, 67, 180, 181
Vitamin C 65
Vitamin D 65, 67
Vitamin E 159
Vitamins 21
  deficiency 24
  folic acid 24, 65
  supplement 64, 65, 66, 180
Von Brandes, Dr. J.W. 6

W
Weight gains 2, 8, 50, 53, 167
Weight loss 5, 34
Wheat 37, 38, 39, 67, 72, 180
Wheat germ 72
Whey 27, 28, 64, 71, 76, 78, 178, 180,
  181, 182
Worms 41

Y
Yams 28, 63, 72
Yeast 9, 10, 13, 24, 26, 47, 54, 57, 64
Yogurt 3, 15, 27, 61, 62, 63, 66, 69,
  71, 74, 155

In Remembrance...

This marks the thirteenth printing of *Breaking the Vicious Cycle: Intestinal Health Through Diet*. At the time of the author's death in September 2005, the book had sold over one million copies and had been translated into seven languages.

Through *Breaking the Vicious Cycle*, Elaine leaves behind a body of work that continues to transform the lives of countless individuals who find health through the Specific Carbohydrate Diet. She tirelessly pursued her scientific research until her death at age 84. Since that time, many dedicated people have taken up where she left off to "get the word out," so others will be helped as they were.

In her latter years, Elaine dedicated her research to the food/brain connection, demonstrating the beneficial effects of the diet for those with Autism Spectrum Disorder. The creation of the Gottschall Autism Center in Massachusetts is one more way that her work and legacy will live on.

"Elaine had so much enthusiasm for life that one thought she must go on forever. Elaine, we all want to say thank you for being you, for what you have done and for your book, which is your legacy that goes on and on helping people."

Pat Nelles, a friend whose daughter was healed by the SCD

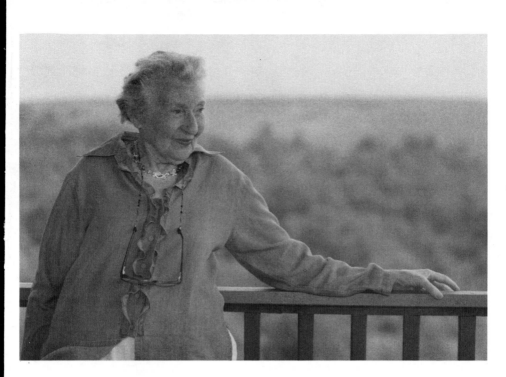

About the Author...

Elaine Gottschall, B.A., M.Sc. received her Bachelor's degree from the Department of Biology at Montclair State College, Montclair, N. J. in 1973 where she graduated Magna Cum Laude. She entered the Department of Graduate Studies in Nutrition at Rutgers, the State University of New Jersey, New Brunswick campus, that same year.

In 1975, Mrs. Gottschall moved to Canada and became a member of the Department of Cell Science at the University of Western Ontario's Zoology Department. She spent four years there investigating the effects of various sugars on the digestive tract, working mainly on the cellular level. She obtained a Master of Science degree in that Department in 1979. Results of her work are published in the journal, *Acta Anatomica* 123:178 (1985).

For the year following, Mrs. Gottschall worked in the Department of Anatomy of the University of Western Ontario investigating the changes that occur in the bowel wall in inflammatory bowel disease.

Her main interests have been the effect of food on the functioning of the digestive tract, as well as on behavior.